THE AUTISM HelpBOOK

SARAH CARRASCO

City Bear Press
Manahawkin, New Jersey

Cover photo of Sarah Carrasco and her son, David by Megan Elizondo.
Cover and book design by Lynn Else

Copyright © 2018 by Sarah Carrasco

Library of Congress Cataloging-in-Publication Data
[to come]
[last line CIP data]

ISBN 978-0-692-14117-5 (paperback)
ISBN 978-0-692-14492-3 (e-book)

Published by City Bear Press
19 Henry Drive
Manahawkin, NJ 08050
www.citybearpress.com

Printed and bound in the
United States of America

This book is dedicated to my son David:

David,

You are a light in this world. Although you have suffered in ways no child ever should, you maintain a sense of optimism that is astounding. You are kind, nice, generous and always fair. Your gentle nature and sense of calm brings peace to our home. Everyone who knows you loves you. I have watched you slip away from me and into the world of autism. By the grace of God, you continue to improve and are coming back to me a little more every day.

It is so nice to hear your voice after all those years of silence.

This book is dedicated to you as it was inspired by you. This was never about me, it was always about you. Your story is one of hope, perseverance and love. Your story deserves to be told. You are proof that miracles can happen. You are a miracle. I am inspired by your positivity and endurance; you are brave beyond measure. Thank you for being such a wonderful son and human being.

You are the light the world so desperately needs. Thank you for bringing light into my life. Your brothers and I love you more than words can say.

CONTENTS

FOREWORD

WHEN MY SON DANIEL was diagnosed with autism in 2000 at the age of 16 months, the world as we knew it vanished. It wasn't just the suddenness of the onset of his symptoms at a year old, but also the whirlwind of medical dogma that accompanied our every thought and decision as we grappled with the diagnosis and all it meant. You see, in the dogma of modern medicine, there is no hope, no cure for autism. With the prevailing treatment model reducible to "don't bother," it is no wonder parents are left bereft as their child and family are handed a theoretical life sentence.

From the resultant grief and anger, a legion of families has forged a new way, a path lit by the shared resolve to find answers. This legion has formed a community of researchers, activists, mentors, practitioners, and even world-renowned scientists who look at autism as treatable, and perhaps even preventable. From the synergy of millions of families actively seeking answers, we have made inroads once considered impossible. Our children are improving, with many going on to full recovery, leading productive lives. My son is one of them.

The devastation that often accompanies an autism diagnosis comes largely from the unknown, especially when traditional medicine dispenses so much advice that is flat-out wrong. Most parents would do anything to help their children if they only knew *what* to do, what steps to take first, and how to continue. Instead, parents are dismissed by medical and therapeutic professionals with platitudes that include phrases like "possible group home" or "might work in the basement." In many cases, we are given the worst possible prognosis for our child's future and sent on our way without even the slightest bit of hope.

With *The Autism Help Book* Sarah Carrasco taps into those early days after her son's diagnosis. She has been in your shoes. So have I. We know the complexities of autism in ways no one can define for you except for those who have gone through it. Sarah takes a street- smart approach to navigating, and implementing, the path forward. It is this simple practicality that encourages parents to take the first steps. What may otherwise be daunting is broken down into small, doable pieces that can catapult parents forward and lead to real changes, especially for their children.

The Autism Help Book focuses first and foremost on the need for parents to take care of themselves in order to best help their children. As a testament to this fact, I landed in the hospital twice in one year due to a stress-related heart condition because of the uncompromising approach I took to helping my son. That tunnel vision, which included the notion that I simply didn't matter as long as my children were okay, was not healthy for any of us in the family. It took two years to reclaim my health, which is why I was pleased to see Sarah proclaim "take care of yourself" in chapter 1. As on the airplane when the oxygen mask drops, the adult needs to place their own mask on first before placing their child's. Same principle applies to autism families. Keeping an eye on our own health, while simultaneously seeking healing for our children, is crucial for the long-term well-being of the whole family.

THE AUTISM PARADIGM HAS SHIFTED

Since my son's diagnosis the autism community has grown in numbers, unfortunately. But we have also grown in knowledge. As a mentor to hundreds of families over the years, I can categorically say the future for children diagnosed today is far better than for those diagnosed a generation ago. The reason for this comes largely from what we have learned about the causes of autism—the genetic pathways involved and their environmental triggers—accompanied by greater knowledge of how to repair the damaged immune system.

My son's recovery from autism by the age of four was considered an anomaly back in 2003. Today he is one of many considered fully or significantly recovered from autism. Mentoring parents these days begins with the goalpost in sight. We know kids are going on to healthier, independent lives. We also know that those earlier prognoses for our children were absurdly wrong. By virtue of the fact that you are reading *The Autism Help Book*, you have taken the first step toward making a bold declaration for your child too. Namely, no one knows the potential of any child...especially yours. So let's set the bar high with a bright future as the goal in sight.

THE PITFALLS ON THIS JOURNEY ARE TEMPORARY

One of the most poignant moments on my journey of helping other autism families was the message I received from Sarah telling me that my 2004 article about my son's recovery from autism played a key role in her ability to find answers for her son. In her message she described how the article saved her son's life. As a fellow parent I read those words with gratitude for that glimpse into our shared heartache. Gratitude because all parents on this journey have a bond that acts as a bandage to get us through the bad days. And there will be plenty of bad days. But from those pivotal moments of pain and anguish in her own life, Sarah

THE AUTISM HELP BOOK

has been able to channel a way forward with resolve and fortitude. You are holding in your hands the virtue from that resolve.

Mary Romaniec
Author *Victory over Autism*, Skyhorse, 2016

INTRODUCTION

Be the change you want to see in the world.

—Unknown but often attributed to
Mahatma Gandhi

I REMEMBER SITTING in my car after working a long, difficult day. I was stuck in traffic in my beat-up 1996 Honda Accord. The AC struggled to churn out semi-cooled air and the car's radio worked only in between bumps in the road. I was hot, stressed, and plagued with worry for my son who has autism. I was also angry. I was angry that my son suffered with what was described as "worst-case scenario for autism." I was angry that my marriage fell apart despite my best efforts to save it. I was angry that I didn't have babysitters. I was angry that people stared at us in public. I was angry that we had no money. I was angry about everything.

As I felt myself being consumed by anger, I forced myself to think of three positive things:

One, my son David was improving every day. He was no longer violent; he was communicating with word cards and was making eye contact. Two, after having been denied for SSI (Supplemental Security Income from the Social Security Administration) twice, a fellow autism parent explained to me how to get approved. Now I could afford more out-of-pocket treatments that were sure to help my son. Three,

---

I had read an article entitled, "Daniel's Success Story: A Determined Mother Demonstrates that Full Recovery from Autism Is Possible," and because of that determined mother, I was starting to get my son back.

These three things helped ease me out of my bad mood. I realized too that I had support from other autism parents. Those brave mothers and fathers who came before me were my greatest asset.

As I simmered down I lifted my head and looked up at the Subaru stopped at the red light in front of me. It was a beautiful sunny day. The sun shone down on the car ahead of me, and the light refracted in rainbow rays. It was so unusual that I was taken aback. To this day I have never again seen sunbeams so distinctly brilliant as at that moment. As I marveled at the beauty of the sun's rays, I looked down at the car's bumper sticker. It read, "*Be the change you want to see in the world.*" In an instant, my anger and self-pity dissolved.

In that pivotal moment I realized that because an autism dad took time out of his day to help me get David approved for SSI (which we desperately needed for his care), David would soon have the insurance he needed for his medical care. It occurred to me that my son's violent behavior had disappeared because an autism mom took time out of her day to write an article that would change the course of our lives. That moment changed how I saw my life with autism. My perspective was changed by something as simple as a bumper sticker. My life didn't have to be all doom and gloom; I could choose to find the silver lining. I could be bitter and angry, or I could be the change I wanted to see in the world.

In that moment, I decided that I, too, would help other families affected by autism. Life with autism can be hard, but what if I could make it just a little bit easier for families? What if I wrote a guidebook for parents who had a child with autism? I would help them with resources, insurance,

Introduction

disability law, special education services, therapy options, special diets, and biomedical interventions. I could be the person I wished I had had with me on my worst days. I could be other autism parents' faraway best friend. I would walk them through the dynamics of changing relationships in the face of an autism diagnosis. I would tell them that it is okay and often necessary to grieve. I would tell them how to pick up the pieces of their lives and make them whole again. I would be the mentor I had so desperately needed. I would be the change I wanted to see in the world.

As the years have gone by, I have actively supported people with autism and their families. I have participated in mentor programs where I worked one-on-one with families affected by autism. I have sat on expert panels for Individualized Education Programs (IEPs) and have worked as an educational advocate for people with autism. In immersing myself in the community, I have now worked with hundreds of parents of children with autism and have identified their greatest areas of need.

I know that I cannot personally reach every family affected by autism. I cannot walk each family through everything they will need to know. The best way for me to communicate all of this to the autism community is with this handbook.

Autism is complex. The therapy and medical interventions are complex. The legal issues are complex. Educational needs and rights are complex. I have done the groundwork and have spent years getting services in place for my child and countless other families. There is no point in you having to suffer through these arduous processes as I did. I have done the hard work and put in diligent effort to ensure my son has the highest quality of life I can provide for him. In order for your child to thrive, which in turn will make your life easier, you will need to know where to start.

This book will give you a place to start. It will provide the thing you need most right now, which is hope. There is hope for your child, for you, and for your family. There is hope of vast improvement and even recovery from autism-related symptoms. There is hope for your finances, for your relationships, and for your future. There is hope, and it starts here.

1

FIRST THINGS FIRST: TAKE CARE OF YOURSELF

Be kind, for everyone you meet is facing a hard battle.

—Ian MacLaren (Rev. John Watson),
a noted Scotsman, author of
Beside the Bonnie Brier Bush

THANK YOU, MR. MCLAREN. You must have known some parents of children with autism. The truth is that we do face a hard battle every day, and until my son David was about four and a half, I literally couldn't go to the mailbox, change his clothes, give him a hug, or feed him without a battle royale. Having a child with autism is complicated to say the least. The time it takes to care for your child—or children—with autism can leave little-to-no time for relationships, play groups, family, or fun. It is an all-consuming endeavor.

That is why taking care of yourself needs to become a priority. You need to be healthy, well rested, and reasonably happy to do a good job in researching and organizing the services your child needs. At first this may appear to be a bit of a "chicken and egg" dilemma since it is nearly impossible to take care of yourself adequately without the support services your child needs in order for you to catch a break.

For example, until recently it was difficult for me to focus on one thing for long because David had to be watched constantly. I have a little one named Brooks, who clearly inherited my Viking genes, and my middle child, Aidan, who needs and deserves my attention after years of giving up his time, so I could care for his brother. I have so much going on during the day that I've learned to make lists to keep myself organized and focused on the task at hand. My best advice when beginning your autism journey is to start by making short lists of realistic goals for the day and coming week. I personally use Post-it Notes and put them on my kitchen cabinet. It's not fancy, but it works. However you choose to keep notes, make lists, and/or create a calendar is entirely up to you. The important thing is that we find creative ways to stay focused, so we can take care of ourselves and our own needs.

Each chapter will provide a short list of topics I will cover that will enable you to get things on the right track. I hope you appreciate lists as much as I do. So here it is, my "to-do" list for chapter 1, and your to-do list as you begin this journey:

- Talk to a local social worker who is knowledge-able about autism services
- Apply for respite care funding
- Find support in the autism community
- Take care of your own health
- Allow yourself time to grieve
- Stop feeling guilty

TALK TO A LOCAL SOCIAL WORKER WHO IS KNOWLEDGEABLE ABOUT AUTISM SERVICES

Your local social worker can help you with some very important questions: Where do I find local resources? Which doctors are the best? What funding is out there? How do I cope with the stress? I was incredibly fortunate to have had a dedicated and knowledgeable school social worker when David was in an autism-specific preschool program. She helped me get organized. She encouraged me to get the ball rolling, and I took it from there—just as you will.

State and county school districts may vary in policy, but all schools have a social worker who is available to you during the school year. School social workers are hired by school districts to enhance the district's ability to meet academic goals. They work to create a cohesive plan of care for the child. They will work with the family and school to ensure the child, family, and school all have access to vital resources. Their job is to aid in academic achievement, but they are also the people who generally know the most about community resources. School social workers are trained to help families access information pertaining to mental health concerns. They offer behavioral support in the classroom and home and will consult with the teacher, administrators, and parents to ensure the best outcome for a child with autism.

If your child is in an autism-center program, typically referred to as an autism spectrum disorder (ASD) classroom, or is in a special-needs program, you may have a social worker who works specifically with the children in these classrooms. If there is no social worker designated for your school's program, you can request a meeting in person or by phone with the general-education social worker to discuss community resources.

I worked as a paraprofessional in special education for two years. During that time, I met several school social workers. Some were on top of their game, some weren't. I learned that if you have a school social worker who is right out of college, he or she might mean well but may have no idea what resources are available.

If you have a special-needs school social worker who seems inexperienced, politely push that person to do the research necessary. If he or she is not responsive to your needs, go to the school social worker. Give him or her time to do some homework (a month, tops), and if you still don't have answers, contact a supervisor. I know that going to someone's boss will not make you any friends. While I believe that "you catch more bees with honey," there are times when I have to put my personal feelings aside and do what's best for my son, whether it makes me popular or not. Sometimes to get results we need to be bold and do things outside our comfort zone—like speaking to a supervisor. Most social workers are great, but again, some of them may need guidance from their superiors in order to help families who are trying to access local resources.

I was blessed to encounter a dedicated school social worker, Mary Curtin. Mary told me about the Developmental Disabilities Resources Center (DDRC), now called A Better Choice (ABC), which is my local community-centered board (CCB). These organizations provide information to parents on federal, state, county, and city disability programs and also manage and disperse funds for many of these services, particularly those funded by Medicaid and/ or Medicaid Waiver programs.

ABC employs resource coordinators who help parents with their children's specific needs. It may be called something different in your county, but every state and county has an organization similar to ABC. In some states, The Arc (formerly the Association for Retarded Citizens, but now known as The Arc) acts as a CCB, while other states offer resource coordination through their Human Services or Social Services office. No matter which agency is designated for this, your school social worker should know exactly whom to call. Not all school social workers are as knowledgeable as mine was, but they should be able to lead you in the right direction with regard to community programs and available funding.

One thing I've had to learn is to never take no for an answer when it comes to my child. Maybe the first social worker you speak with will not have the answers to your questions, but there is one who does. Winston Churchill, in a speech given in 1941, is often paraphrased as saying, "Never give up." While I love this quote, it is inaccurate. What he really said was "Never give in. Never, never, never, never—in nothing great or small, large or petty—never give in except to convictions of honor and good sense. Never yield to force; never yield to the apparently overwhelming might of the enemy."[1] Whether we are paraphrasing or not, the message remains the same. Never give up! There is always someone who has the answers to your questions. You just have to keep asking until you get the right person. Never give in, never give up!

There are several avenues to pursue to find helpful, knowledgeable social workers. If your child has medical needs and you are in and out of hospitals, contact the hospital social worker. That person should know of programs and resources in your area and can help you access the paperwork needed for services.

Another option is to contact your local health department and ask for a social worker who can advise you on community resources. Many parents need behavioral support for their child, and the health department should provide a social worker who can refer you to an organization similar to Colorado's CCBs and guide you to appropriate behavioral support counsel. I recommend that parents start with a school social worker, but the health department is always an option and a good backup.

The symptoms of autism vary significantly from person to person. Some children with autism do not require intense behavioral support, while others need it on a regular basis. The health department should be able to provide contact information for social workers who can guide you toward resources pertaining to developmental disabilities and direct support for families affected by autism.

My son's autism manifested itself with violent outbursts that were severe enough that I skipped "Door Number 1" (the health department) and went straight for "Door Number 2," the mental health department. I explained that I could not easily take David out in public and could not bring him in for behavioral support meetings. They said, "No problem," and sent an LCSW to my house the following week.

What is an LCSW you ask? Good question. It took me a couple years to figure that one out myself. An LCSW is a licensed clinical social worker. My LCSW, Karen Hardison, was sent to my house for behavioral support.

I will never forget that first visit. Poor Karen. David was going berserk when she got to the house. He was in the bedroom (actually, my parent's guest bedroom as we had just moved back in with them—awesome, I know), and he was going for the "Most Destructive Toddler" world title.

In the forty minutes Karen was with us that day, David broke four pictures that were on the wall (except the picture of Jesus and Mary, whom he refers to as Jesus's mommy) and tore the blinds down in the guest room. He ran to my parents' room and pushed their TV off its stand. Karen and I ran in the room and saw the TV on the ground. As soon as we got to my parents' room, he took off back to the guest room and pushed the guest room television off the dresser. BOOM! Two TVs and four pictures down in less than a minute.

Karen and I spent most of the visit keeping David from hurting himself and picking up glass. I hated for anyone but me to see him in that state of mind, but I was also glad she was there to witness it firsthand. I needed her to know how serious his behavior was and how desperately I needed behavioral support for him.

Karen came to the house two times a week for the first six months. At that point David was nonverbal, so she spent most of her time supporting me in my parenting of David. Karen helped me realize that David's behavior was not my fault and that I was doing everything I could for him. She was right; I *was* doing everything I could to help him. The sad thing is that no one had ever said that to me before she did! She told me that I was a good mother and that I was doing all the right things.

Just as importantly, Karen was nice to me. She was one of the only people at that time—the worst time of my life—who was truly nice to me. As it turns out that was all I needed. I just needed someone to say something positive to me, about me, so that I could feel happy again, if even just for a moment.

Karen was so encouraging. She was always happy to see David and me, a response I was not accustomed to at that time. She gave me lists of local agencies that dealt with autism, and she also gave me lists of improvements David had made and improvements I had made as a mother. Karen was all about lists and I love lists, so we were like two peas in a pod. She and Mary Curtin, David's school ASD social worker, epitomize what good social workers should be: They should be helpful, they should have meticulous notes on local resources, and they should always be a source of encouragement to parents of children with disabilities.

I know that I just dropped a ton of information on you, but I want to emphasize the importance of taking care of yourself, and the best way to do so is to locate the right resources and professional support as quickly as possible.

For a while it may seem that the only people in your support network are skilled professionals. When things are really tough, that may just be exactly what you and your child need. An ordinary friend may be too overwhelmed! You may not need more than one social worker, as I did. You may just need the ASD social worker to help you get the resources you need.

I have included several types of social workers so you know that there are options for you. They are there to support you and your child. Keep looking until you find one who seems genuinely interested in the needs of your family. Social workers are, generally speaking, exceptionally good people and are available to you in many different facets of life. Just ask around, and eventually you'll find the one you are looking for.

APPLY FOR RESPITE CARE FUNDING AND WAIVERS THAT PAY FOR RESPITE CARE

It is very important that you locate your state's version of a CCB before searching out respite care. They are often designated by county or, if there are many small counties near each other, they may be grouped together. Either way, your state's human services department should know how to connect you with developmental disability (DD) resource centers. Human services departments will have access to DD councils who oversee funding and programs for kids with developmental disabilities (or delays).

Contacting human services may be your best option for getting connected to DD resources in your state and/ or county. These organizations will have access to support groups, therapy providers, respite-care providers etc.

Respite care is probably one of the most important aspects of taking care of yourself. Someone at ABC asked me if I wanted to apply for respite care funding. My response was the ever-impressive blank stare. I literally had no idea what they meant by respite care. They had to explain that respite care funding is another way of saying, "money to pay a babysitter." I was like, "Yes! Sign me up for that right away!" I didn't have the resources to pay anyone a decent amount of money to watch my boys, and I knew this might be the only way I would be able to do so. Although applying for respite care can happen at any time, it is a crucial first step for many parents who desperately need a break.

When you are the caregiver of someone with autism, it is essential to get a break once in a while. It does not mean you don't love your child or that you are not coping. It's just a part of being human.

Getting out of the house is essential for parents of children with autism. We need a break from the monotony and a chance to reconnect with who we were before our lives got turned upside down. It's not irresponsible or neglectful to leave your child with a skilled person who knows how to take care of him or her while you take a break. It's self-preservation.

Getting back to the subject, there are a variety of avenues to pursue respite care funds. The Autism Society in your state can help you find out which organizations or government programs are available to access respite-care funding. You can find a local Autism Society chapter or affiliate at www.autism-society.org. Most states have an Autism Society affiliate, but if yours does not, you can contact The Arc at www.thearc.org. Your social worker may also have contact numbers in your area or know of programs that are applicable.

The Arc is great about supporting parents with respect to services and resources. In Colorado The Arc offers a class called "Mobilizing Families," which is a three-part course that explains various resources in Colorado. The information shared in the class covers respite care funding, how to apply for a Medicaid Waiver (more on this in chapter 3), summer camps for children with disabilities, and more.

Parent to Parent is another good organization. It has programs in most states and can be found at www.p2pusa. org. Parent to Parent is an online support group of parents, as the name suggests, designed for parents to share information on autism and other disabilities. Again, this is not in every state, but if it is in yours, make contact and ask the online group where to apply for respite-care funds.

There are a number of ways to access information on respite care, but again, you may only need that initial meeting with the school social worker to pinpoint where and how to apply for funding. It is the necessary component in getting some reprieve from the day-to-day stress.

As an endnote to this section, I want you to know two important pieces of information your disability resource center should tell you. One, your child is eligible to have diapers paid for by Medicaid once they are over the age of four. Two, the income guidelines for families who have a child with a disability in the house are much higher than for those families who have all typical children. If your resource coordinator does not tell you these things, they may not know the job very well. I, apparently, was eligible for food stamps for years, but because my resource coordinator wrongly told me there was no income difference, we had many years where I chose between paying bills and buying food. If you are told there is no difference in income for food stamps (now called food assistance), reach out to your state agency that deals with income guidelines for food assistance.

FIND SUPPORT IN THE
AUTISM COMMUNITY

Parenting a child with autism is different for every person, but for me, one of the hardest things is the feeling of isolation. I feel isolated from every person I know at times, and it helps me to be among people who are in a situation similar to mine, people who have knowledge of and insight into autism.

The Autism Society, The Arc, and Parent to Parent are great places to connect with other parents of children with disabilities. I realize that not everyone has access to the Internet, but you can find these organizations locally by phone. Support groups give you someone to talk to who has had similar experiences and can empathize with you and your situation. I have found that other parents are often the greatest source of information. Parents can tell you which doctors are helpful, which therapies have worked, where to go for play groups, and what resources are available in your area.

One of the most important things I have learned is to sift through information and advice people give me on autism. I am constantly getting advice on what I should do to help David from family, friends, day care workers, and even random people at the park. Some advice is helpful, but the majority of advice I receive is redundant and, quite frankly, annoying. Although they mean well, most people I meet do not have history with autism. They do not know how to support me or David, and they simply can't relate to the complexity that comes with raising my son. I have learned to separate fact from opinion and to follow my own path in choosing what is, or is not, best for my son. Remember, you are the person who knows your child best!

In addition to filtering out the excess advice, it is important that you find a place where you feel welcome. I don't know about you, but I feel like an outsider almost every place I go. People stare at David and me in the store, the doctor's office, the mall, restaurants—pretty much everywhere. I feel like an outsider in my own family at times. Don't get me wrong; most of the people in my family are amazing. My family is, in general, kind, and they don't pass judgment on us.

But no matter how kind or understanding they are, my family members still don't know what it's like to raise a child with autism. They don't understand that I can't always sit down and have a conversation with them. They may not comprehend how difficult it is to sit down and write out Christmas cards or send out family pictures. My life is so different from theirs that it makes me feel strange and even foreign among the people who are closest to me.

The only way to remedy this feeling is to socialize with people with whom we *can* relate. The Autism Society of Colorado has family events a few times a year where I can bring David. No one stares at us. They are unmoved when he flaps his little hands, and they don't stop the conversation to stare when he spins in circles. They know that it is just part of having autism, and they don't fault us for it. It's a relief to have that one place to go where my son and I can feel just like everyone else.

Finding ways to socialize is important, but we all have different needs when it comes to this type of thing. I was more comfortable finding one or two parents to connect with than I was attending a support group. Having few babysitters, the thought of going to a weekly meeting gives me a panic attack. For me, and again every person has different ideas of the support they need, I do better with small groups or one-on-one interactions. Other people are more comfortable belonging to a support group, and some of them are great. I should warn you, though, I have been in some groups where the majority sit in silence while one or two parents go on and on about their experiences.

The groups to look for are the ones that have a mediator who monitors time and who can keep the parents focused. Mediated support groups are more productive and topic-specific than groups that allow for belly-aching. Mediators can keep the group focused on the topic of the week, be it sibling support, finding a dentist for your child with autism, or any of a number of other issues. A focused support group will prove to be more beneficial than an open-ended gab session.

If you are not able to find a support group that interests you or cannot attend meetings regularly, or, if you are like me, then finding another parent who can relate to you may be the more suitable option. It might take a while to find someone you click with, but it's worth the effort to have a friend you feel comfortable telling the ins and outs of your days to. Besides, most of us parents of kids with autism have epic poo tales of either diarrhea or constipation. We need one another; who else is going to listen intently to that kind of story?

TAKE CARE OF YOUR OWN HEALTH

I should start by saying that the idea of writing this book was something I had reservations about. I knew that the only way to help other parents was to, in part, tell my story. I am a private person, and I tend to keep things of a personal nature to myself. However, a while back I heard a man give his testimony at church. He told of his life prior to finding God and everything in between. I realized then that we should share our stories, not to bring attention to ourselves, but rather to shed light on the journey we must all make toward an enlightened and peaceful life. I learned that we share our stories to benefit others and not necessarily ourselves.

Although I would not bring up the following in casual conversation, I think it is important to share this part of my story with other parents of children with autism. So here it goes: Through all the hardship—my divorce, medical bills piling up, a bankruptcy (immediately following le divorce), family who had no knowledge of autism, a career that was put on hold—I neglected to take care of myself. This eventually led to fibromyalgia.

Fibromyalgia is, from what I understand, directly linked to stress and depression. I don't remember feeling depressed for long periods of time, but I was stressed beyond the limits of what my body could handle. I was also sleep deprived. David has had issues with sleep and wandering, and I haven't slept well his entire life as a result. The lack of sleep coupled with the stress I was experiencing was an assault on my immune system, and eventually my body broke down.

It got to a point where I could no longer pick up my children. I couldn't sleep because I was in too much pain. I had a hard time walking, and I was no longer able to keep up with housework.

Having no insurance, I was reluctant to go to the doctor, but after a month of the undeniably bad state of my physical health, I made an appointment. Luckily, I saw a physician's assistant (PA) who had done his master's thesis on fibromyalgia. He knew right away what was wrong with me and advised me that there were drugs for the disorder and that he thought healthy eating and exercise could improve my symptoms.

I went from his office to the bookstore and bought *Reversing Fibromyalgia*, by Dr. Joe M. Elrod. The book recommended a 21-day detox diet which included mostly organic fruits and vegetables and excluded all of the junk food I'd been eating as a matter of convenience. It recommended an exercise program and a list of vitamins that are essential to good health. I did most of the things in the book and am happy to report that I have never felt better.

The point is this: I was so stressed out and overwhelmed that I allowed my body to deteriorate. I should have been taking good care of my physical health, but I was so bombarded by everything around me that I became the last person on my list of priorities.

In retrospect there is not much I could have done to avoid most of the stress I was under, but I could have handled it differently. I could have eaten better, and I could have stopped myself from thinking negative thoughts night and day. *What will happen to David when he is an adult? Where can I find a decent babysitter? How can I afford to put Aidan in sports?* These and other questions plagued me night after night. Did I find the answers to my questions by 2 a.m.? No. Was eating junk food my only option? No. I set myself up for disaster, and fibromyalgia was the end result, a disaster.

I could have looked at having fibromyalgia in a negative way, but I really think it was a wake-up call. Some might say it was nature's way of telling me to slow down. I say it was God's way of telling me that it was time to start taking care of myself.

We do no justice to the world we live in by giving too much of ourselves. If we are worn down and unhappy, what good are we really doing for the people around us? When David was at his worst, I rarely left his side. I had convinced myself that my staying with him every moment would somehow help him get better and prove to everyone that I was trying everything I could to care for him. It was a ridiculous notion but, nonetheless, a notion I held on to for many years.

Once I started getting out and socializing again, I felt better. I felt like me again. I never understood the expression, "you can't see the forest for the trees", until I had time to reflect on the years I had spent refusing to leave David's side. It basically just wore me out. It ran me down and gave me no opportunities to do any research on autism or to meet people who could help him.

Looking back I realize that I had actually done him a disservice by not getting out and looking for answers. I had done him a disservice by not keeping myself happy and healthy. No one wants a mom who is worn down and cranky, including kids with autism.

When you have a child with autism, it is hard to get out of the house for a variety of reasons, but if you have some-one you trust to watch your child, put this book down and go! Get out and do something *you* want to do.

My favorite thing to do is hang out with my friends and do nothing. It's like that episode of Seinfeld when Jerry and George are pitching their idea for a show to NBC. They explain that it is a show about nothing.[2] That is exactly what my friends and I do, an intentional, inexpensive, noth-ing! We pretty much all have kids, so when we do hang out, we're all too tired to party like rock stars. We just watch movies or listen to music. It's not exciting, but it makes me happy to sit down for more than five minutes. It makes me happy to feel like me once in a while.

Even when you are in the house with your child or, in my case, children, it is possible to still take care of your-self. If you love music, listen to music. If you like to dance, dance in your living room. If you like to paint, paint in between your super-exciting household duties. Find a way to be happy again. You deserve it, and your child deserves to have a parent who has a good disposition.

Another way to take care of yourself is to eat healthier. I dreaded going on a healthy diet, but after a month on the diet, I felt much happier. I had more energy and I was sleeping better. I heard once that anything you do for 30 days becomes a habit, so try it out for a month. If you feel better, stick with it. I also avoided eating healthier because I thought it would be expensive.

As it turns out, it really isn't all that much different in cost from the junk I used to eat. I buy organic bananas, spinach, carrots, and healthy cereal. These four foods are the staple of my diet. They are convenient and inexpensive, just my kind of thing.

Don't kill me, but exercise is important too. David was so hard to take care of for so long that I couldn't exercise. Taking him on a walk was not an option. Leaving him at the day care center at my gym was not going to happen. It's not always easy to find time to exercise, but when you are able, exercise is a great way to release endorphins. It will increase your energy levels and it makes you look better, which never hurt anyone.

One thing that differentiates parents of children with autism from other parents is that we need to have flexibility in our jobs. In addition to needing time off for the inevitable—kids getting colds, dental appointments, yearly check-ups, etc.—we need time off if our child is having a meltdown at school. We need time off for school meetings and time to observe our child in the classroom at least once a school year. We have therapists to hire and insurance companies to deal with. Many of us need to have some flexibility at work in order to make sure that our child is getting the services they need.

If you have an incredibly stressful job or you work at a place that has no flexibility, look for a new job. Start sending out resumes or ask people you know if their employer is looking for help. Visualize or even make a list of the qualities you would find in the perfect job, and keep looking until you find it. We have enough stress—we don't need to add a crappy job to the list! Finding a new position may also come with fringe benefits. It may offer more paid time off or better insurance. Remember, it can't hurt to try!

A great way to get a break is to befriend another parent of a child with autism. If it is someone you see as trustworthy and competent, you can take turns babysitting one another's children. It is the only way a lot of parents get a break, and it will also give you the opportunity to get free childcare! It helps me more than anything to have other moms of children with autism as friends. It's a relief to not have to explain David's behavior every five seconds, and it's great to have someone watch him every once in a while.

ALLOW YOURSELF TIME TO GRIEVE

I'm not saying it's easy to be happy when your child has autism. I'm not saying that it will be simple to find a babysitter so that you can go out and seize the day. What I am saying is that it's okay for you to be happy. There is no shame in your enjoying life. Before I came to peace with the diagnosis, I went through a long and substantial grieving period. I didn't cry about it much, but when I did, it was a deep and sorrowful cry—the type of cry that scares you because you can't catch your breath, the cry of a mother whose child suffers profoundly. I cried once in a great while. In part my tears were attributable to stress and a lack of sleep, but mainly I cried out of grief.

I, like many, if not most, parents of children with autism, went through a grieving period. I grieved for David's pain and his inability to tell me he was in pain. I grieved for the time he lost playing with other children and his inability to play with me. I grieved for my parents because it was hard for them too. I grieved for myself and the hardship I had endured fighting with doctors, nurses, and insurance companies.

I allowed myself to feel the grief that was tugging at me *all the time.* It is important to allow yourself time to grieve. There is no shame in it. You need time to accept the diagnosis and time to be sad once in a while. It can be sad, and pretending it isn't won't help anyone, including your child.

I still have days when it hits me like a ton of bricks. I am still adjusting, but I am rarely consumed by the grief. It's just part of my life now. It is emotionally healthy to see things for what they are and then find a way to make the best of it.

That is really what I want to convey: I want other parents to know that it's okay to feel that sadness for a while, but it passes. The grieving process is undeniably hard and it is continuous, but it is of the utmost importance that you allow yourself time to grieve. It is not weak. You are not feeling sorry for yourself. You are not taking on the role of a victim. You are not wrong to grieve. It is the hardest thing I've ever had to accept.

I spent many years telling myself that it would all go away, that this isn't happening, that David's symptoms would suddenly disappear. I was in denial for a long time, partly because I didn't want him to suffer and partly because I knew the emotions that were sure to come with the diagnosis would be sharp and brutally painful. But it wasn't until I accepted the diagnosis and grieved that I was able to really accept him for the awesome little man that he is.

The truth is that David is one of my favorite people in the world. He is pure, innocent, and sweet; he is an example of how people *should* be. It wasn't until I accepted the diagnosis of autism and allowed myself time to grieve that I really appreciated David. He is amazing and is just perfect the way he is.

I always loved him, but I was so confused by his behavior and almost offended by his lack of affection toward me. I was angry that I couldn't go out in public with him. I was mad that no one would babysit him. I was angry because for me it is easier to be angry than it is to be sad. Anger is a cheap and readily available emotion. It is sadness and grief that are hard to face and even more difficult to endure.

Once I accepted that my son did have autism, that he was going to be different from other kids, I started to see the upside. I recognized how clever and interesting he is, how smart he is, and how loving he can be. Grieving gave me the opportunity to come to terms with the sadness and anger. It opened my eyes to how devastated he must feel. It was grief that gave me insight into his world, a world I am now a part of.

It was the grieving period that made me realize that I am the luckiest woman in the world to have a son who is different from the rest of us. He is better than me. He is more compassionate and brave than I will ever be. Grieving gave me the opportunity to realize the truth, and the truth is that he is my rock, when all this time I thought I was his.

Grieving, and accepting, the diagnosis of autism gave me the chance to have a relationship with my son other than as his caregiver. It was grief that pushed me out of my self-pity and into a new frame of mind. Grief was the real emotion I felt, not anger, not pride, but grief. It was the emotion that put the diagnosis in perspective, and it was the turning point in my life as well as David's life. It can be the hardest emotion we face, but it is also one of the most profound. It is the only way to accept things for what they really are instead of what we want them to be.

I also think it is good for parents to read Jenny McCarthy's book, *Louder Than Words*.[3] It helped me to hear a parent talk about the funny side of autism. Although it can be incredibly hard on us, our kids do funny things, and it's nice to be reminded to laugh once in a while. I should note, however, that one autism mama I recommended this book to said, "There are too many curse words." I personally don't mind the language, but in case you do, fair warning: She drops a lot of f-bombs (but I still love her).

While I realize that life with autism can be hard—really hard—there are certain things parents do to make life with autism harder than it needs to be. When you've been doing this as long as I have, you see the difference attitude makes in a child's life. The attitude, negative or positive, will always impact the child with autism.

While I know it is hard to be positive every day, it's important to keep things in perspective and to appreciate how hard it would be to live in a world where you cannot speak but you understand everything that goes on around you. People with autism are people, with feelings and emotions, no different from the rest of us. They need our love and approval just as much as a typical child does, maybe even more. I think, until a parent has allowed themselves time to grieve, it is impossible to have a chipper attitude or to even recognize what a child with autism is experiencing.

Allowing yourself time to grieve and accepting your little guy, or girl, for who they are, is the key to moving on. Grieve until you can't anymore. Cry until you can't anymore. Scream, hit pillows, do whatever you have to do to get those emotions out. It's time to move on and get the joy back in your life. It starts right now, with you giving yourself the "go-ahead" to grieve.

STOP FEELING GUILTY

Over the years I have met many parents of kids with autism. The one reoccurring theme is that we all feel guilty about something. One might feel guilty because she hasn't yet taken her child to see a dentist. Another feels badly because she has no time for her friends. Another parent is disappointed in himself because he can't spend enough time with his kids. As good parents, we care and we strive to be better—two admirable qualities. However, we can only do so much. We all have pangs of guilt, but it isn't always the appropriate emotion.

My guilt came in the form of blaming myself for David having autism. I was plagued with thoughts of inadequacy. Had I not eaten the right foods when I was pregnant? Was I responsible for his autism because I allowed people and circumstances to stress me out when I was pregnant? Was it my obsessive-compulsive cleaning, hence exposure to toxic chemicals, during my pregnancy that led to him having autism? Was this my fault? I felt guilty because it was the only thing left to feel. All of the emotions that I expected to have as a mother had gone out the window and what was left was grief and guilt. Guilt won out as the lesser evil.

I continued to blame myself because doctors kept telling me that they didn't know what was wrong with him. I told at least five of the pediatricians I took him to that I thought it was autism. They said I was wrong. One doctor eloquently described him as a "brat" and said that I should discipline him more. How insightful.

I blamed myself until I went to a pharmacology clinic at my community-centered board, A Better Choice (ABC). I requested the pharmacology clinic at the urging of David's school social worker. The purpose of the clinic is to determine if a child needs to be medicated for behavioral issues.

The pharmacology clinic was made up of a panel of specialists: a child psychologist, a child psychiatrist, a behavioral therapist, David's resource coordinator at ABC, and his school social worker. They wanted all medical records and as I sorted through the hundred and forty pages of records, I noticed something. Every time he received a vaccination his symptoms had increased. His two-week shots marked the first day of what his doctor referred to as "colic." He cried at least 10 hours a day and his tummy was hard as a rock. Six months, thirteen months, eighteen months, two years, all his vaccinations were followed by a trip to the doctor where I explained that he seemed more distant, his bowel movements were irregular, he cried more, slept less, spoke less, and ate less.

I felt guilty until then because it wasn't until then that I realized that it wasn't *me* who had caused his autism. Before you start beating yourself up, go over your child's medical records. Request them from the doctors you've seen if you no longer have copies (you have a legal right to all medical records that pertain to your minor child).

I don't mean to go off in another direction. I am smart enough to know that the vaccine-autism connection is controversial. I am not trying to raise controversy; I am trying to relay my empathy for those of you who are riddled by feelings of guilt. We tend to blame ourselves even when we've done everything within our power to provide a good life for our kids, which often includes having them vaccinated.

So back to the pharmacology clinic: Several different pediatricians had previously recommended that I put David on anti-psychotic medication, and two professionals at that meeting told me I should consider "out-of-home placement." He was between three and four years old when the recommendations were made. I refused to fill the prescriptions or send him to "a home" without a proper diagnosis. Only then would I let the pharmacology clinic help me decide if medication was an appropriate choice. It turns out that the main thing, the huge thing, that the clinic helped me with was my guilt as it got me to review David's medical records.

As I said before, there was a six-month gap from the time I signed up for the clinic and the actual appointment date. Every professional in the room had read David's medical history. The paperwork they had reflected a child who was violent, self-injurious, nonverbal, and at risk of hurting himself or others.

The child that came to the meeting with me that day was a much different David than the one they had record of. I had taken him in for allergy testing, and he'd tested positive for peanut, soy, rice, and oat. In addition to removing the foods he was allergic to from his diet, I put him on the gluten-free/casein-free diet. The dietary changes alone made him a completely different kid. Addressing the food allergies and diet subsequently addressed the behaviors.

We, as a group, decided that David did not need anti-psychotic medication, nor did he need any other type of behavior meds. Since the behaviors had decreased, it was quite evident that he did not need to be placed "out of the home." What he needed was for me to pay attention to his symptoms and to take the initiative to move forward with dietary changes.

Up until that time I always felt guilty, as if I weren't doing enough, and I know that many parents feel the same way. When our children are not well or are unhappy, we tend to put the blame on ourselves when, truthfully, there may be an underlying cause we have not yet thought of. Going over your child's medical records and taking a closer look at what has worked for other parents of kids with autism is a good place to start.

We face a hard battle on a daily basis, all the while feeling guilty for things we can't control. In all honesty, most of us give 100% every day, and there is nothing to feel guilty about when you are doing the best you can. From one parent to another, don't make the mistakes I've made. Love yourself for the effort you've made thus far and for the mountains you will climb tomorrow.

If I can leave you with some insight, it would be to say that it is okay to learn from others' mistakes, mine in particular. Take a break once in a while, take care of yourself, and grieve if you feel like it. Don't think you need to have it all figured out today, and never be afraid to ask questions (even if you feel stupid asking). Don't feel guilty for the past or for the things you cannot do. Just move forward.

I think that what overwhelms parents is when they start thinking about the word "autism." If that word and the implications that come with it overwhelm you, don't think about the autism. Instead, focus on the child and how much they love you and need you to stay strong. Our kids can and do get better, but it starts with us being able to take care of ourselves and to stay positive in our thinking.

Having given myself license to grieve, to get healthy, and to get the right support, I took my life back. I chose to focus on David and his potential rather than the diagnosis of autism and everything that comes with it. I chose to put my family above all things (except for God), and I chose to move forward.

As Plato said, "Be kind, for everyone you meet is facing a hard battle." Keep in mind that this applies to you as well. Be kind to yourself.

NOTES FOR CHAPTER 1

Note to readers: I am adding a blank page at the end of each chapter for parents to take relevant notes. Again, I wrote the book I needed in the beginning of my autism journey. In the beginning, our life was hectic, and I lost many of the notes, email addresses and phone numbers that I needed to get us organized. My hope is that these extra pages will give you a place to take notes pertaining to the chapter and help you keep everything together.

2

TAKE THE NEXT FIRST STEP: GETTING THE DIAGNOSIS OF AUTISM

If you're going through hell, just keep going.

—John Randall Dunn

AUTISM ON A BAD DAY can look a lot like hell. Ask anyone who has been kicked, hit, spit on, and screamed at, all while cleaning up broken glass or smeared feces.

Our lives, as honorable as they may be, are difficult. We, in the midst of our hell, must keep going. We have no choice. I remember feeling hopeless when David was first diagnosed with autism at the age of four. My family's life—more specifically, David's life—is so much better now than it was when we received the diagnosis. I write this book from the perspective of where we were then and what it took to get us where we are today.

This chapter will offer information on how to cope with and understand your child's diagnosis. Again, one thing I've found to be helpful in my life with autism is to make lists. So here is my to-do list for getting a diagnosis of autism:

- Recognize the symptoms of autism
- Make an appointment to see a specialist

- Understand the autism spectrum
- Organize your paperwork

Many parents know that their child has autism well before they receive a formal diagnosis. Each one of us comes to this realization in our own unique way. There are always telltale signs that your child may have autism spectrum disorder (ASD). Although each one of us has our own story of how we received the diagnosis, we are bound by a common thread: The diagnosis can be devastating, and it is life changing.

Although the diagnosis of autism may be upsetting, there is hope. Most kids with autism can make vast improvements if they start therapy (also called early interventions) and biomedical interventions (more on that in chapter 4) at a young age. In addition to that many of our kids can achieve more appropriate social behaviors as they get older. It seems that no one ever tells you that in the beginning, and I wish they would.

David started out as being labeled "severely autistic." He is now happy, communicates verbally, and he is affectionate. In the beginning, it may seem as if your child will stay stuck forever in the place they are in now, suspended indefinitely in their own private world. I can assure you, though, that parents who put forth effort dedicated to their child's well-being can yield amazing results. No matter how "severe" the autism may be, there is always hope.

In the beginning it is natural to feel panicked, overwhelmed, and uneasy about the road ahead. If you are in this phase, please know that it is just that—a phase—and like any phase, it will pass. This time of your life is what I call *in medias res,* which is Latin for "in the middle of things." I learned this phrase in college and for whatever reason, it stuck with me when David was at his worst. I would tell myself that I was in the middle of it all and someday things would be better. I wish I had known years ago that David would one day be happy and speaking, but while *in medias res,* it's hard to imagine your life ever being restored. Your life, believe it or not, can be happy and peaceful again. When it's all said and done, you will be strong beyond measure and, like us veterans, you will know what it is to have a steel spine.

I remember in great detail how difficult our life was around the time David was diagnosed with autism. It took years to get a diagnosis, and when I found out he did in fact have autism, I was alone. It was just me. My thoughts were racing. After seeing almost every specialist I could find in Colorado, I sat at my father's computer and typed "no language, no eye contact, does not catch a ball" into the Google toolbar. Immediately, a myriad of autism websites came up.

As I sat there reading symptom after symptom that were exact descriptions of my son's symptoms, I felt an impending doom seeping out from deep inside my soul. The words "there is no cure" popped up on the screen. That moment will be suspended in my memory for the rest of my life. I remember how I felt—as if every piece of me hurt. I read those words, stood up, and knocked the heavy leather office chair over with a loud THUD. As quickly as I was brought to my feet by the words "there is no cure," was as quickly as I was brought to my knees. For the first time in my life, I was involuntarily brought to my knees, consumed by grief.

My knees hit the floor and soon I was on all fours in a feeble attempt to catch my breath, crying so hard I was unable to breathe, choking and gasping for air. I have never cried so hard in my life. A million thoughts ran through my mind. I was twenty-seven years old and my marriage had already fallen apart. I had no one to talk to who would understand; I had no money, and no support system. The thoughts that crippled me, rendering it impossible for me to stand, were of David. What would happen to him? Would he go to college? Get married? Would he ever speak? Would he ever tell me he loved me? A selfish thought at the time, but it was one of the hardest things for me as a mother. I just wanted my son to say he loved me.

I was engulfed by the emotions that were brought out by one little word: autism. If I had known then that at age 16 David would be hilarious, smart, witty, and happy, I probably would have taken the news a bit better. But I didn't. I didn't know that there *was* hope for kids with autism because the website said (I don't even remember which site it was), "there is no cure," and I just couldn't get past that.

Therein lies the problem, there is plenty of hope and help for our kids, but we are not told that at the moment we recognize our child has autism or at the time of diagnosis. Google doesn't have a pop-up that reads, "Hey! You there! Everything is going to be okay. You just have to find the right resources."

When our child is finally diagnosed we are told that they have a lifelong disorder for which there is no cure. We are sent on our way, our hope and will dissipating as we leave the doctor's office to begin our new life, a life with autism.

Every parent responds differently to the diagnosis. For me, it was the absence of hope that diminished my will and crippled my ability to move forward. At the time, I was still playing the, "who can diagnose him?" game, taking him to specialist after specialist until, finally, the bottom dropped out.

I took David to a pediatrician who had been in practice for 25 years. After reading the symptoms of autism online, I was convinced that David did in fact have autism. She specialized in kids who had a variety of disabilities. I took him to see her with the highest of hopes. I thought, *She'll know what to do; after all, she has 25 years of experience under her belt!*

When we got to her office, David, as usual, brought the house down. He was screaming, crying, and kicking anyone who dared come close to him. After 20 minutes of glares from other parents and the office staff, we were taken back to a room.

The doctor came in and observed him in his usual state: David was still screaming and would not, under any circumstances, allow her or the nurse to take his weight, temperature, or any vitals for that matter. She looked at me, wide eyed (*Uh-oh*, I thought, *She's a deer in headlights—she won't be able to diagnose him*), and said, "What are we seeing David for today?"

I said, "Obviously, something is going on with him, and I don't know what it is. I need a diagnosis for him." With David screaming and dismantling the room, she said, "Have you tried anti-psychotic medication yet?"

With tears welling up in my eyes I said, "He's four years old. I'm not doing that. I just want to know what's wrong." Her response was, "Medication is something you should consider to give yourself a break."

"Look," I said, "I was told to come see you because you've been in practice 25 years; I know you can help us. I think it could be autism." She said, and I will never forget this, "In 25 years I have never seen anything like this, and you'd better hope it's not autism because, if it is, it's the worst case I've ever seen."

Ouch.

I left that appointment demoralized and even more broken-hearted than I had been before I went in. It was, however, a defining moment: It was the moment I realized that no doctor could help us. Knowing what I know now, I understand why no one could diagnose him. It was hard to pinpoint exactly what was going on with David because his autism was so severe that it would be next to impossible to diagnose him based on past precedent. In her defense, she was right. In all of my years of research, I have only seen one video clip of someone as severely affected by autism as my son.

The following month David had occupational therapy with a certified occupational therapist assistant (COTA) named Cindy who brought me an article that would change our lives forever. The article was called "Daniel's Success

Story: A Determined Mother Demonstrates that Full recovery from Autism Is Possible," by Mary Romaniec.[1]

That was my first glimmer of hope in four years. No one had ever told me that recovery was possible or that it was even an option. I remember sitting outside my house reading the article; I was happy for the first time in years. It was as if God Himself had sat down beside me. The sun shone down on me with perfect warmth, and a cool breeze hit my shoulders; it was true peace. The weight I had carried for so many years was gone in an instant. I had the one thing I needed to survive: hope.

I realize that you, too, may need hope as badly as I did. So here it is, from one parent to another: There is hope. And, yes, my son is getting better every day. He no longer hits, kicks, or screams in pain for seemingly no reason. He makes little jokes, sits for haircuts, and keeps up with his weekly chores. Coming from the "worst case" of autism, I think he's doing quite well.

It is important to reiterate that without that hope it would have been impossible for me to get him better, feeling as I did that I had no place to start. Hope that he would someday be happy is what drove me. Hope is all that it took for me to climb out of the pit of despair and snap back to reality.

There is hope. Just keep reading; everything will come together.

Chances are good the word *recovery* is all that you hear right now, and that is wonderful. Recovery is possible, not in every case but in many cases. And if full recovery does not happen, vast improvement can.

As much as I'd like to continue on this topic, it is for another chapter. For now, the focus needs to be on getting a diagnosis of autism for your child so that you can get the right therapies in place immediately. Recovery is possible, but the diagnosis comes first. So, let's get to it!

RECOGNIZE THE SYMPTOMS OF AUTISM

Recognizing the symptoms of autism is paramount in your decision-making process. Some children have a speech delay but do not have autism. Others may exhibit poor impulse control and are not meeting their developmental milestones, but they do not have autism. Some may have violent outbursts accompanied by poor social skills, but they do not have autism.

Autism is unique in that diagnosing it requires a specialist with a trained eye, but it also requires that a number of criteria are met in order to make the diagnosis. I have observed many children on the spectrum, and from experience I can tell you that there are certain indicators that parents must look for. There are always signs that your child has autism. Many of these signs are subtle at first but should be taken seriously if they don't start to resolve themselves by the time your child is about three years old.

Please note that this list of autism symptoms is not clinical or exhaustive. There are plenty of medical references for clinical diagnostic criteria. This list is mine; a list of symptoms that I've seen in countless children, each of whom had a resultant diagnosis of autism.

Social

1. Little-to-no eye contact
2. Disinterest in other children/a preference to play alone
3. Lack of empathy or inability to understand the emotions of others
4. Little-to-no interest in bonding with parents or other family members
5. Lack of response to facial cues or nonverbal communication

Sensory

1. Heightened sensory response to noise, touch, visual stimulus, or smells
2. An acute response to activities of daily living (ADL's) such as brushing teeth, combing hair, changing clothes, bathing, etc.
3. Sensory issues with eating, which can include avoidance of certain textures or gagging when introduced to a new food
4. Hand flapping, spinning, rocking, and/or clapping
5. Seeking the sensory stimulus of pressure, such as wanting to be hugged or squeezed tightly, burrowing self under a pile of heavy blankets, stuffed animals, or pillows

Communication

1. Total lack of speech
2. Regression in speech ("Timmy used to talk all day; now he only says 'hi.'")
3. Significant delay in language development compared to peers
4. Repetition of words or echoing words they hear (echolalia)
5. Little self-generated, spontaneous, or conversational language
6. Inability to answer questions in a meaningful way
7. Responds to questions with one or two words as opposed to sentences
8. Poor pronunciation or articulation of sounds
9. If verbal, fixation on one topic and will not deviate from the subject

Behavioral

1. Throwing frequent tantrums or seems easily agitated
2. Screaming or crying frequently and without apparent cause
3. Flailing arms, hitting, kicking, biting, pinching, etc. on a regular basis
4. Unusual play, such as lining toys up rather than playing with them, spinning wheels on a car but not rolling the car on the ground, separating toys by color or size but not playing with them, stacking toys, etc.
5. Appearing withdrawn with preference to be alone

Again, autism manifests itself differently in every child. The lists I've provided are symptoms I've encountered over the years and are often indicators of ASD. There are varying degrees of symptoms and behaviors, but there are always commonalities among our kids. The commonalities are what aid doctors and specialists in making a diagnosis of autism. If your child has several of the symptoms listed above, it is time to contact your pediatrician.

MAKE AN APPOINTMENT TO SEE A SPECIALIST

If you believe that your child may have autism, there are some necessary steps you must take in order to get a diagnosis. Some private insurance companies, and even Medicaid, require a referral from your pediatrician in order to cover the cost of "specialist" care. Other insurance companies, such as Kaiser, do not need a referral, and parents can set up specialist appointments on their own. Check with your insurance company, and if a referral is required, you can call, fax, or email your pediatrician's office and ask for a referral to a developmental pediatrician, or ask the office who they use to make autism diagnoses.

You will most likely see a developmental pediatrician or a developmental psychiatrist. Your primary doctor will guide you toward a specialist in your area. Doctors don't all use the same formula for diagnosing autism. Pediatricians use a variety of diagnostic tools to assess where your child is developmentally. Some may use what is called (CHAT) which is short for *Ch*ecklist for *A*utism in *T*oddlers. Others may use the *A*utism *D*iagnostic *O*bservation *S*chedule, or ADOS. No matter how the doctor or specialist comes to the conclusion that your child has autism, there will most likely be paperwork involved, so try to get to the appointment early and bring someone (helpful) with you if possible.

There are specialists in the mental health field who can make a diagnosis of autism. One example would be a child psychiatrist; this person may reference what is called the *D*iagnostic and *S*tatistical *M*anual of Mental Disorders (DSM) in order to make a diagnosis of autism. It is now referred to as DSM-V as it is the fifth edition. Diagnostic labels are used to pinpoint a specific medical condition. With autism there will always be substantial delays in social skills which, in part, justify the diagnosis of autism.

Although the DSM-V provides diagnostic criteria, I believe that autism should not be listed in it because autism is not a mental health disorder. In my opinion autism is neurological and biological and is not an issue of mental health at all. The fact that autism is listed under the DSM is indicative of how far behind we are in terms of autism research; we aren't even classifying it correctly.

There are many ways to go about getting a diagnosis, but one of my favorite organizations is the *A*utism *R*esearch *I*nstitute (ARI). They offer what is called the E-2 checklist which parents can print out and return. It is a diagnostic tool and is helpful for parents and doctors as well. The checklist asks a variety of questions about your child. You can mail it in and get feedback from the experts, or you can fill it out and see if you feel it gives you direction. This is not a formal diagnosis, but it can be used by parents to determine whether or not they need to pursue additional developmental testing for their child. You can access the E-2 checklist on the ARI website, autism.com, at the URL listed in the notes at the end of the book.[2]

In addition to getting a diagnosis of autism, your pediatrician or specialist may want your child to undergo further testing. It is common for our kids to have genetic testing to rule out any abnormalities that could be causing autism-like symptoms. You will most likely be given referrals to additional specialists. The protocol is the same for each specialist appointment. Depending on your insurance, you will most likely need to hang onto the written referral and fax or email it to the insurance company in order for them to cover the cost of the visit.

There may be certain circumstances in which your pediatrician will suggest a CT (computerized tomography) scan, MRI (magnetic resonance imaging), or an x-ray. Although this is somewhat uncommon, it may come up at some point in your child's life. For us, David had a *huge* bump on his head as an infant. When he was five months old, I took him to have an x-ray of his skull. He screamed and kicked the entire time, but we were able to get the x-ray after several attempts to keep him still. Although they found nothing, his pediatrician had told me that some babies have water retention on their skulls after birth. It made no sense to me (still doesn't), but the point is that these tests may come up if your doctor feels there is good reason for them.

The reason many parents, including myself, choose to go through with x-ray, CT or MRI testing is to make sure there are no major issues with the brain or a possible fracture of the skull. If there is in fact scarring on the brain, for example, the scarring may be affecting speech and language, and the symptoms can look a lot like autism.

Although you may not want to put your child through any more testing, it is important that you rule out any other possible causes for their symptoms. Many illnesses can look like autism and the reason these additional tests are important is to determine if, in fact, there are underlying health issues which are causing autism-like symptoms.

Your pediatrician may also recommend blood work, hearing screens, or psychiatric evaluations to rule out any additional concerns he or she may have. I agree with most of the testing because there are times when children display autism-like symptoms when they may only have a hearing deficit, for example. There are cases when children are diagnosed with autism and later their parents find out that there were issues with brain swelling or scarring. There are logical reasons to go through these tests. However, don't feel pressured to do everything at once.

Testing for physical and genetic concerns is incredibly difficult for parents and, of course, the child. Spacing visits out is probably the best approach. I do think that we, as parents, have an obligation to do everything we can for our child. I do not, however, think that our kids should be test subjects. It is our job as parents to find the happy medium between gathering important medical information and inflicting unnecessary discomfort and possible trauma on the child.

As a parent you will make your first empowered decisions after receiving the diagnosis of autism. Which tests do you follow through with and when? You are the one who has to get your child with autism bathed, dressed, fed, and out the door—kicking and screaming, in all likelihood—to go to the doctor's visits. You can prioritize the testing and do what you feel is most important first. I suggest following through with genetic testing as soon as you can because this test can indicate disorders that can look a lot like autism but may be another medical issue entirely. It is rare that this testing will lead you to a diagnosis other than autism, but I feel that it is important to rule out genetic concerns while the child is still young.

Genetic testing is becoming more popular in the autism world. Many parents are choosing the 23andMe test which allows them to look at raw data pertaining to the child's genetic profile. It is also common to look at *methylene tetra-hydrofolate reductase* (MTHFR) mutations as well. Dr. Amy Yasko wrote a book, *Autism: Pathways to Recovery*. The book is about genetic mutations which can affect methylation, a function of the body that enables detoxification. More on that in chapter 4.[3]

David has had every type of medical exam and test you can think of. It was really hard on him to be held down or strapped down to have blood work or x-rays done on his little body. It sucked. He would scream and cry through the entire visit, every visit. On top of that, the doctor's staff would often fall apart on me. During our visits they were often visibly shaken, sometimes in tears. It was obvious that they had no training or experience with severe cases of autism. The professionals were of no comfort to me or my child. In fact, their inability to hold it together would elicit a negative response from David. He is very intuitive, and when the nurses and doctors were agitated, he recognized it and would escalate the behavior.

As parents it can be very frustrating to go to these appointments when medical personnel have not been properly trained. It is important that we find ways to cope when we are in these difficult situations. You may have a Bible verse or perhaps an inspirational quote that motivates you to stay positive. I would recommend writing down your favorite quote and taking it with you. Trust me, it helps.

In order for specialist visits to be productive, someone has to remain calm. I often found myself being the only person in the room who could hold it together. It got to the point where I had a little script. When I would see the staff starting to fall apart, I would say, "I live with this 24 hours a day. All I'm asking for is 15 minutes. If you do that, we'll be out the door and you can go on with your day." It usually worked because it put things into perspective for them.

As a mother I shouldn't have to be a counselor at doctors' visits, but this is an example of what it takes to be successful in your child's autism treatment. You have to do things that are outside of your comfort zone for the sake of your child. Sooner or later you will find yourself doing things you didn't know you were capable of. You'll be a super-mom or dad in no time flat.

There are also the unconventional methods of getting a diagnosis of autism. In some cases I've had parents tell me that they have never had their child formally diagnosed; rather, they put their faith in the school system to do so. In these instances, parents noticed early on (under the age of three) that their child was not reaching their developmental milestones and contacted their local preschool for help.

Preschools will administer developmental testing to indicate where the child is in relation to peers of the same age. In most cases preschools will use a Vineland assessment tool. The Vineland assessment tool is used to establish patterns in social, personal, behavioral, communication, motor, and daily living skills. It is often used in schools because it helps the teachers and staff to establish how to best meet the needs of your child.

In addition to the usual methods of obtaining a diagnosis, you can always track down a *Defeat Autism Now* (DAN!) doctor, or what is now called a MAPS doctor (*Medical Academy of Pediatric Special* Needs). If you want to learn more about these doctors, you can go to the MAPS website for more information (the URL is in the notes at the end of the book). You can click on the tab labeled "Clinician Directory" to find a doctor near you if you are interested.[4] However, generally speaking, I would go to another specialist before seeing a MAPS doctor because specialist visits are usually covered by insurance and MAPS doctors are typically out of pocket. Genetic testing, allergy testing (I suggest doing blood work, not a *skin prick test*, or SPT), and other blood work should be covered by your insurance provider.

David's pediatrician recommended that we see a psychologist or a psychiatrist for an evaluation. The pharmacology clinic we went to had both a child psychologist and psychiatrist, but again, by the time David saw them, he did not need behavior meds. I do not think that my child needs a psychiatrist or a psychologist, despite what I was told years ago. He was violent for so many years because he was in pain and because he could not tell me he was in pain. The only means of communication he had was behavior. His behavior indicated that he didn't feel well, not that he needed behavior medications at age four. Addressing his allergies and removing gluten and casein, for example, decreased the unwelcome behaviors by 90% because he was no longer in pain.

David's food allergies were so severe that his stomach most likely hurt day and night. He would often hold his head or bang it against the ground, probably from headaches caused by the allergies. His seasonal allergies surely gave him a sore throat, and his eyes were constantly red and irritated. He clearly did not feel well but could not express that to me. No mental health professional could have helped him with the behaviors because they were physiological, and David's physiological needs had to be addressed before the behaviors would decrease.

Again, you as the parent should feel confident in your decision-making abilities and need to approach the suggested medical testing in the way you see fit. Prioritize which appointments should come first and stick to your plan. It is you, after all, who has to bear the burden of getting your child there and paying for the visit.

After the appointment with the specialist who said, "You'd better hope it's not autism because if it is, it's the worst case I've ever seen," I realized that I needed to take a new approach. I was on my own and needed to find answers from people who had walked in my shoes. In my case, I literally was on my own as well; soon after that visit, my ex-husband told me that he had cheated on me when David was 10 months old. Fabulous.

Although I wanted to forgive him and keep my family together, I just couldn't get over it. I filed for divorce soon after he told me the news. Raising David and his brother, who was one at the time, wasn't easy, but it got even harder when their dad moved out of state and we didn't see him for a couple years.

At the time, I had a picture of Eleanor Roosevelt taped to my wall. The picture was of her pulling a suitcase behind her. The quote below read "You must do the thing you think you cannot do." During that time, I remember (on several different occasions) looking at David, who was a million miles away. It occurred to me that even though I didn't think I could raise him on my own, I had to. I had to do the one thing I didn't think that I could do. I had to raise a child with special needs and a one-year-old with no financial or emotional support.

There were days when I wanted to fall apart, but with David being so severe and me being on my own, it was hardly an option. I managed to keep a smile on my face and act as if everything was okay, even though I was broken inside. In a way it's probably a good thing that I didn't have the option of falling apart, or I surely would have lain in bed all day, crushed by the weight of my reality.

This may sound cheesy, but one thing that helped me to cope with David's autism was the book *The Secret*, by Rhonda Byrne. After reading this book, it made me more mindful of how I was thinking about our life, and I started to think about David getting better and someday going to college. I also stopped feeling sorry for myself and started feeling sorry for David instead. It was he, after all, who was actually going through hell and not me. *The Secret,* gave me a new perspective on autism. It helped me to see that my son is amazing and that together he and I can get through the bad days if I stay positive and maintain a sense of optimism about our future.

I still have days where I slip back into negative thinking, but in general, I now stay focused on the positive things in our life. I stay focused on him getting better and all of the amazing improvements he's made. If and when you struggle to see the positive side of your life with autism, find an inspirational book to get you back on track or, at least, be mindful of your thoughts. They are more powerful than we often give them credit for.

By the time David was formally diagnosed at age four, I was pulling myself together and was thinking a bit more positively. After careful research helped me clarify the autism diagnosis, I called David's pediatrician and asked for a referral to a doctor who specialized in autism. He referred us to Children's Hospital here in Denver. But there was a catch: We had to wait six months to be seen.

After six long months we went to our appointment. I wasn't expecting sage-like advice or resource referrals; all I wanted was a diagnosis. When we got to the appointment, the doctor was waiting for us. He and two residents observed David for a few minutes, and after they quietly discussed my child, he walked up to me and said, "What are you here for today?"

I said, "I think he has autism, and I want to know what you think."

He responded eloquently by saying, "Of course he has autism. What do you want from me?"

At this point I was so used to people treating us poorly that I didn't miss a beat. I said, "Nice. I just need a diagnostic code of 299.00 for insurance and school purposes. I also want recommendations for behavior therapy, OT [occupational therapy], and speech. When can you have that in the mail?" He agreed with the recommendations and promised to have the written diagnosis to me in a timely manner. After a short discussion on diet, David and I went on our way.

Getting the diagnosis the way I did was horrible, but even under perfect circumstances—a loving spouse, a supportive family, and having money in the bank—there is no easy way to hear that your child has autism. It hurts. There is no other way to say it.

UNDERSTAND THE AUTISM SPECTRUM

When David was first diagnosed, I felt overwhelmed in every way. One overwhelming aspect of the diagnosis was all of the acronyms that were coming at me: *OT, IEP, ABA, PT, SLP, IDEA, ADA, ASD. Are these people speaking a different language?* I had no idea what all the acronyms meant, and I'm sure they are mind-boggling to some of you as well. Fear not, dear reader, I've provided a list of acronyms in chapter 6! It took me a while to figure this all out, but the hardest to grasp was ASD. What in the world does ASD mean, and what does it mean to my family?

According to the American Psychiatric Association:

> People with ASD tend to have communication deficits, such as responding inappropriately in conversations, misreading nonverbal interactions, or having difficulty building friendships appropriate to their age. In addition, people with ASD may be overly dependent on routines, highly sensitive to changes in their environment, or intensely focused on inappropriate items. Again, the symptoms of people with ASD will fall on a continuum, with some individuals showing mild symptoms and others having much more severe symptoms.[5]

There it is, the clinical definition. It is useful to clinicians but doesn't really help us as parents to understand where our child is on the spectrum. ASD reflects all kids who have some form of autism, but our kids are individuals and, as such, we must determine where each is on the spectrum.

People with high-functioning autism are often said to have Asperger syndrome, which, in a nutshell, means they have language and they can care for themselves in regard to daily living skills but will have poor or (at best) awkward social skills. A well-known person with Asperger's is Dr. Temple Grandin. Dr. Grandin has autism and is able to live an independent and amazingly impressive life. She has a Ph.D. in Animal Science and is an Associate Professor at Colorado State University. She has designed livestock-handling facilities that are commonly used in the U.S. and is a lecturer on ASD.

Temple Grandin is wonderful. Her book *Thinking in Pictures* helped me to understand David in a way I never would have on my own. She explains things from her perspective, the perspective of someone with autism. It is clearly important for mothers and fathers to bond with their children, but when you have a child with sensory issues, hugging and kissing them is often impossible. She not only explains why bonding is difficult, she offers her own solution as well: she created a squeeze machine that helped her to feel centered and calm when she was on sensory overload.

Not being able to hold your child is something many parents of children with autism experience. The lack of physical contact can be detrimental to bonding with your child. I could never really hold David for long, and he didn't seem to want to be hugged. I didn't understand why until he was about five years old and I read *Thinking in Pictures*. Here's what Temple Grandin says in her book about sensory issues as they relate to autism:

> From as far back as I can remember, I always hated to be hugged. I wanted to experience the good feeling of being hugged, but it was just too over-

whelming. It was like a great, all-engulfing tidal wave of stimulation, and I reacted like a wild animal. Being touched triggered flight; it flipped my circuit breaker. I was over-loaded and would have to escape, often jerking away suddenly.[6]

There it is: our kids want to be hugged and loved just like every other child, but hugging often triggers a sensory response that makes them feel completely overwhelmed. She explains that as a child, she would seek pressure by lying under sofa cushions or wrapping herself up in blankets. She also says that the need for "pressure was biological." This explanation of sensory-seeking behavior helped me to understand how to help David when he became overwhelmed, and it also helped me to bond with him a little better.

I like her books because it gives us, as parents, insight into our children's minds, a place we are rarely allowed. Temple Grandin reflects one end of the autism spectrum, and while she thinks in pictures, not all people with autism do. Although high-functioning autism or Asperger syndrome is the best-case scenario for autism, make no mistake, it is incredibly hard to live in a world where you feel socially isolated. Getting your child in a support group for children with Asperger's can be very beneficial to them in the long run.

The relevance of knowing where your child lands on the spectrum is important when it comes to which therapies you will pursue. If your child has Asperger's, for example, seeking social skills groups and behavioral therapy is the best approach.

On the opposite end of the spectrum are people like my son when he was four. People on this end of the spectrum are typically nonverbal or have very limited language. They cannot live independently. They do not appear to be learning in school (although this is often misleading). They may be violent, have a tendency to wander off, or lack safety awareness, and will be socially withdrawn.

Again, David's autism was so severe I can't begin to compare it to anything I've read about or even heard of. If we're talking about severe cases or low-functioning autism, it would look a lot like David in years past. His symptoms manifested themselves with violence toward me and those around him. He would kick us and bite us. He escaped from day care, bit day care workers, and was kicked out of several centers. He screamed, broke lamps, televisions, and toys, tore up papers, books, and money. He was the opposite of Asperger's. He had, as the doctor said, "worst-case scenario for autism."

In between these two ends of the spectrum, there are a myriad of possibilities. You will see sensory issues that vary in severity. There may be speech issues, social skills deficits and/or learning delays.

If your child is given a diagnosis of PDD, PDD/NOS or Rett syndrome, they are on the spectrum but meet certain criteria in order to get that diagnosis. PDD is yet another acronym which means pervasive developmental disorder (PDD). With PDD, there are notable delays in social skills, imaginative play, and fine motor skills. In PDD/NOS, the NOS means "not otherwise specified." When you have the NOS added to the diagnosis, that typically means that the autism is mild, and that there are minor social skill delays. Rett syndrome is defined by a lack of social skills with a physical component. Children with Rett syndrome will have difficulties with coordination and will struggle with motor skills.

Some children with ASD may receive a diagnosis of *childhood disintegrative disorder.* This typically means that the child has social impairments and will need support in the areas of motor skills, age appropriate play, and social interaction.

The significance of the spectrum is that it tells us, as parents, what therapies and services our children need. For example, a child with Rett syndrome will probably need a physical therapist, an occupational therapist, and may need a social-skills play group. It is possible that they may need a speech therapist as well. If a child has high-functioning Asperger's, they will need help establishing appropriate social skills but may not need any additional therapies.

In the long run, your child will benefit from the diagnosis if the corresponding and recommended therapies are implemented. The autism spectrum is very broad, and I could write an entire book on this subject alone, but for now getting the diagnosis of ASD is the focus. Once that is in place, you can take the recommendations of the specialist and start to look at resources specific to your child's place on the spectrum.

ORGANIZE YOUR PAPERWORK

I remember what life was like before David started getting better. It was chaotic and I could barely get through the day, let alone stay organized. Although you may not want to add anything to your hectic schedule, it is vital that you keep all of your child's paperwork and medical documents organized.

You will need to have easy access to all of your paperwork for many reasons. Insurance companies will need documentation from a medical doctor or therapist in order to approve therapy or subsequent medical treatment. If you apply for Medicaid, you will need to have the diagnosis and doctors' notes readily available.

Another reason you will need to have your paperwork handy is for school purposes. If your child is on the spectrum, they may need to be in an autism-center program in school or they could need to be pulled from class for speech or occupational therapy. The school your child attends should ask you for any medical history that applies to your child. Doctors' notes, therapists' recommendations, and developmental evaluations are useful tools for schools and can be used to help them create a program based on *your* child's needs. The more knowledge the school has about your child, the better they can serve him or her.

There are a few easy ways to keep all of the paperwork together. You can do the good old "pick a drawer" and just put any and every document that applies to your child's medical history in there. While this option is not ideal, it is practical, and hey, at least you know where everything is!

One option is to choose a file drawer or buy a file folder (get the large one, you'll need it) and keep all documents in categories. Using a file drawer is effective and will establish a system that is easy to maintain.

The best option is the medical notebook. This option is best because you may need to take your child's medical records with you to appointments. Putting this together is not rocket science, but it takes time and effort to create something that will work well for your needs. Your child, like mine, is an individual and, as such, will have files that reflect their individual medical history.

You will create file folders or categories for a medical notebook based on your child's diagnosis and individual needs. For example, David's files include Applied Behavioral Analysis (ABA), Allergies/Asthma, Behavioral Evaluations, Biomedical Interventions, Diagnosis, Diet, Education, Insurance, Medical Evaluations, Speech Therapy, and Occupational Therapy. In all honesty, his medical file is huge, and although it's daunting to look at, it is necessary to have all of his medical and educational history in one place. I need to reference his paperwork for school and insurance purposes from time to time and it's a lifesaver to have everything handy.

Having a medical notebook will help you feel a sense of security. It is truly freeing to have easy access to everything you may need for doctors' appointments, school, and therapies. It can also help you to recognize patterns in your child's autism symptoms when you look at the records in order by date, including immunization records. Looking at your child's medical file in order can also help pinpoint the onset and severity of symptoms and/or any regressions, such as loss of speech, regression in play skills, loss of eye contact, or increased sensitivity to sound or touch.

I know this all seems a bit overwhelming, but in truth, getting the diagnosis of autism is just the first step in helping your child get the services they need and deserve. It is a life-changing diagnosis, but it does not have to be a lifelong diagnosis. Children with autism recover all the time. It takes work, but it is possible, and everything you've done (or will do) after reading this chapter will set the groundwork for you to gauge where your child is on the autism spectrum, how to treat their symptoms, and how to give your child the best possible autism treatment plan.

A diagnosis of autism is not a bad thing. Parents *not* being told there is hope of recovery from autism, a reduction in symptoms, and that our kids can lead happy and healthy lives—*that* is a bad thing, not autism. In my own life, I can say truthfully that where David was when we received the diagnosis and where he is today are vastly different ends of the autism spectrum. He is no longer violent. He's happy, funny, and patient. He's easy to be around; he likes everything. He's the best brother ever, a wonderful son, and an overall great little man. He is amazing, and I'm honored to be his mother.

The diagnosis of autism is only hard in the absence of hope, and I am here to tell you there is hope—and I'll walk you through it each step of the way. Getting a formal diagnosis is just one step in your child's journey, a step toward healing. While the diagnosis can be devastating for some, and autism, severe autism especially, can be rough on a bad day, remember that, "*if you're going through hell, just keep going.*"[7] Everything will come together in the years to come. Just keep going.

NOTES FOR CHAPTER 2

3

UNDERSTANDING HEALTH INSURANCE AND MEDICAID

Don't judge each day by the harvest you reap but by the seeds you plant.

—Robert Louis Stevenson

IT IS IMPORTANT for parents to stay positive through this arduous phase of our lives. Finding the right health insurance for your child is vital to your family's well-being. You will not have it all figured out overnight. The goal for now is to plant seeds, knowing the harvest is coming in the months ahead.

When I was sorting out insurance for David, I likened it to the movie *The NeverEnding Story*. At times, I felt like I would never figure it out, but eventually it all came together. The seeds I planted eight years ago have indeed brought a harvest! By finding the right health insurance, I was able to help him get to where he is today. I am now getting to know my son, something that seemed impossible in the early years. He is now one of the best and most well-adjusted people I know. Seriously. I always knew he was in there, but it took the right therapy, the right health insurance, and perseverance to get him well.

There is always a logical order in which to do things. First, as we talked about in chapter 1, it is of the utmost importance that you take steps to care for yourself. Secondly, obtaining the diagnosis of autism will help you lay the groundwork for choosing treatments for your child. The next logical step is to start the process of either obtaining insurance, obtaining better insurance, or getting the most out of the coverage you have.

There are several options when it comes to health insurance for children with autism. My son David has had both private and government/state (Medicaid) insurance. One is really no better than the other unless your child qualifies for a waiver, but we'll get to that. For now you just need coverage.

As I said earlier lists are a great way to stay focused in our world. So here it is, the list of things you'll need to know about when it comes to health insurance:

- Private insurance
- Social Security and Medicaid
- Medicaid waivers
- EPSDT
- Autism resources in your state
- The Affordable Care Act

PRIVATE INSURANCE

If you have private insurance, you will have to take the dreaded step of reading the insurance manual you were given when you qualified for benefits. Some benefit packages can be accessed online if you don't have a paper copy. Regardless, you will need to know the basics before moving forward with evaluations and therapy.

There are obvious needs for health insurance: a sprained ankle, stitches (especially for those of us with all boys), etc. But kids with autism need insurance for an entirely different purpose. Our kids need early interventions such as speech, behavior, and occupational therapies. In order to access these therapies (covered in chapter 5), you will first need to clarify which ones are covered by your policy.

It is important that your child receive early intervention services. The younger the child is when treatment begins, the better. Younger children are easier to teach and are less set in their ways. Autism is synonymous with a need for order and routine. If a child does not receive therapy at a young age, it becomes increasingly difficult to change behaviors as the child becomes set in his or her routines.

There is a YouTube video called *Autistic Girl Expresses Unimaginable Intelligence* about a girl named Carly Fleischmann who received intensive behavioral therapy for most of her life. The video was made when she was 14 years old. She began communicating when she was 11 through the use of a computer.[1]

One day during therapy, Carly ran to a computer and typed "help" and "hurt." Several minutes later, she vomited. This was a child who didn't speak and hadn't yet used the computer to communicate. In the months following this momentous event, she was asked to type words in order to go places, get a snack or the like.

If she had not received early intervention services, her progress may have looked very different. She needed an occupational therapist in order to enhance the fine motor skills needed to type. She needed speech therapy to learn not only the alphabet, but the power of language and communication as well.

This child is an example of why we work so hard as parents. She epitomizes the need for sacrifice and dedication from the parent(s). Even though it may appear therapy is having no effect on the child, there are many cases in which the person with autism has actually been retaining everything around them, they just didn't have a way to communicate. Carly's situation is very similar to that of my son's. I was told David would never speak or write, but he can now do both. Carly's parents were told something similar, and look at her now: She is blogging; has a Twitter account (@ CarlysVoice); has interviewed Channing Tatum for her You-Tube channel, *Speechless with Carly Fleischman*; and at the time the story came out, was writing a novel.

It's okay to have hope. It's okay for us to dig our heels in and make a decision that our child can communicate and make progress despite the obstacles in front of them. With dedication, the right therapies, and interventions, our kids can achieve amazing things. It is, however, expensive to get the right therapies in place. For this reason, it is important that the insurance piece be figured out as quickly as possible.

Dealing with insurance companies or Medicaid can be frustrating, but always keep in mind that frustration passes and there is a payoff down the road. Imagine getting to know your child. It may be something that we as parents can barely conceive of, but it is possible. There are steps you must take in order for this to happen. One of these is the meticulous completion of the paperwork needed by your insurance company.

Some companies are amazing when it comes to covering autism-related therapies, and some are not. If your insurance company gives you a hard time regarding coverage of therapies, you will need to write a *letter of medical necessity*. Most insurance companies are now required to fund autism-related therapies, but if your child needs more than they approve, or if you are on a self-funded plan, you may need to write this particular letter.

You can also contact Parent to Parent in your area and see if they have any helpful tips. (You can find them at p2pusa.org to find a branch near you.) Each insurance company is a bit different and each state has different guidelines, so it's helpful to reach out to people in your area who have experience with these companies and regulations. When an insurance company tells me no, I look at it as a jumping-off point. They may think the answer is no; I think,

I need to keep digging until I find a way to justify medical necessity. Keep digging.[2]

If you choose to write a letter of medical necessity, you can use the URL provided in the endnotes[3] or simply Google "sample letters of medical necessity" and choose a template that works best for your child's needs. Writing this letter requires that you have your paperwork handy. You will need your child's diagnosis and any relevant paperwork or documents from pediatricians recommending therapy. For example, if your child was diagnosed by a developmental pediatrician who recommended 30 hours of behavioral therapy and 5 hours of occupational therapy (OT) per week, you'll want to have that documentation on hand.

You will also need to contact your child's pediatrician and explain that you need a letter of medical necessity for (specific) therapy. In addition to contacting your pediatrician, you will also want letters from professionals who work with your child; these can be therapists, home health aides, doctors and teachers.

The letters you are requesting from professionals who work with your child will detail the reasons why therapy is beneficial to your child's development and the impact it will have on them in the years to come. In many cases, if our kids get early intervention services, they can live more independent lives. When our kids live independently, able to maintain jobs and care for their own basic needs, insurance companies actually save money. It is in the best interest of insurance companies to fund therapies for children with autism in the long run. Your job is to help your insurance company see how these therapies and interventions will benefit *them* down the road. Typically, with the right justification, insurance companies will fund necessary treatments.

Writing these letters can be a bit intimidating. Most of us don't write professional-type letters on a regular basis, so if you need help writing or editing your letter, reach out to a family member or someone who can edit for you. We all need a helping hand here and there. Don't feel bad asking for help. The person you're asking may actually enjoy doing it! I love writing, and for someone like me, editing can be fun.

When writing a letter of medical necessity, be mindful of the perspective of the insurance company. Their goal is to treat people in the most cost-effective way possible. Everything in your letter comes down to two things: Is it medically necessary? And will the therapy or intervention save the company money in the long run? With that in mind, it is important to use the correct format and language. Below is a list of helpful tips for writing your letter.

Things to include:

1. Insurance company name and address
2. Your name and address
3. Child's date of birth
4. Diagnosis or diagnoses
5. Therapy or medical equipment requested
6. Length of time therapy or equipment is needed
7. Long-term benefits of medical intervention (e.g., "Speech therapy will increase child's ability to communicate and therefore will have increased opportunities to learn social and vocational [work] skills in an educational setting. These skills can be used in a workplace setting and will allow for little Timmy to seek gainful employment and independent work skills as an adult.")
8. Letters from pediatricians, therapists, schools, etc. recommending specific therapy or equipment
9. Research-based articles, charts, or graphs that demonstrate the benefits of the therapy or equipment requested

Use the words "medically necessary," "research-based," "doctor-recommended," "cost-effective," "promoting independence" and "preventing secondary health concerns." The letter is meant to justify a medical intervention that will help the child gain independence; write from that perspective. As hard as it is, keep it short and focused.

Some states have passed laws mandating that insurance companies cover autism-related therapies. The American Speech-Language-Hearing Association (ASHA) website lists the states that require private insurance companies to cover autism-related therapies. The site is very informative as it includes the many states which have passed this legislation and the maximum benefit amounts for therapy. You can find the URL in the endnotes.[4]

If you or your spouse is in the Military, you may have Tricare as your insurance provider. Tricare's In this case, you will want to access resources through Special Programs. Special Programs, a division of Tricare, provides ABA for children who are diagnosed with ASD. Their website provides information on which autism related services are offered.

SOCIAL SECURITY AND MEDICAID

If, however, you do not have private health insurance, or your insurance provider does not cover autism-related treatment, you will need to apply for Medicaid.

There are many misconceptions about Medicaid. For example, I thought that Medicaid was strictly income-based. I learned, after my ex-husband and I separated, you don't necessarily qualify for Medicaid if you have low income. At the time, I had a part-time job at the time, and even though I only made about $1,200 a month, it was too high an income for a family of three to receive insurance benefits through Medicaid. We had no food, and the little bit of food we did have, I gave to my kids first. I had gotten so skinny

I could see my ribs through my clothes, and even then—so poor I couldn't eat—we did not qualify for benefits.

Sadly, although we did qualify for food stamps, the worker assigned to my case did not return my calls for six months and David's behavior was too severe for me to take him out in public to go to the food stamp office (I took him once and it was disastrous). I couldn't reach anyone on the phone and couldn't get any supervisors to call me back.

It was a terrible time in our lives. David would scream and cry most of the day. He bit, kicked, hit, and scratched me every day. I couldn't even open the front door to get the mail without him having a cataclysmic meltdown.

We had nothing, no resources, no property, and still... we did not qualify for Medicaid. I know firsthand how hard this phase can be. I know there are issues with the Affordable Care Act (ACA), but it does two monumental things for people with autism: It raises the income guidelines for Medicaid so more kids with autism can access insurance, and it forbids an insurance company from denying care based on a pre-existing condition. When David was little and at his worst, no insurance provider would cover him. They pretty much all excluded people with pre-existing conditions. The changes implemented under the ACA are actually hugely beneficial to people with autism. It opened the door for children who were previously uninsurable.

Due to the changes under the ACA, parents now have two options for coverage if they are low-income. The first option is Medicaid (or other state-funded healthcare programs) based on income. This type of Medicaid is useful for covering doctors' visits, dental appointments, and limited therapies. The other option for low-income families is Supplemental Security Income (SSI). SSI covers far more than income-based Medicaid. It was designed to provide income and adequate medical care for people with disabilities.

Now let's get down to brass tacks: A diagnosis of autism should be accompanied by a diagnostic code. These codes vary based on the severity of the autism; in other words, the code reflects where your child lands on the autism spectrum. These codes are essential when applying for SSI.

Those of us who have children with autism diagnosed before October of 2015 will have the diagnostic codes of 299.00, 299.8, etc. If your child was diagnosed after October of 2015, you will use the new codes for autism which will be F84.0 and so forth, depending on where your child lands on the spectrum. The codes are determined by something called the *I*nternational *C*lassification of *D*isease, or ICD for short (again, autism is not a disease, it is a developmental disorder, and classifying it as a disease indicates how little the medical community knows about our kids). The new codes are classified under ICD-10. Again, the codes are simply for doctors, therapists, and insurance companies to communicate with each other about the child's medical history and relevant treatments.

A diagnostic code of 299.00 (or F84.0) can actually be beneficial when it comes to applying for SSI. Diagnostic codes of 299.00 or F84.0 indicate that a child has symptoms that are chronic and will need medical and/or therapy-based interventions. The diagnosis and diagnostic codes can help determine if your child is eligible for Social Security benefits. Diagnostic codes of 299.00 and F84.0 do not guarantee eligibility but may help expedite the process.

Qualifications for SSI are twofold: The child must have a diagnosis (accompanied by a diagnostic code or codes) that meets criteria for a federally recognized disability and must fall under the income cap. The link provided at the end of the book will be a valuable tool in establishing if your child qualifies for SSI based on family income. I recommend reviewing the chart to determine if your child is eligible before moving forward with the awesome task of applying for SSI benefits. The link also provides financial parameters by state, it is important parents know the requirements of their state.[5]

After reviewing the chart for SSI Income Guidelines, you can go online or to a Social Security office to apply for benefits. You can find information at www.ssa.gov, click on the SSI tab and locate the application for "A Child with a Disability." This website allows you to apply for benefits. If you are not sure what you need in order to complete the application, you can check out their "Starter Kit," which outlines the various information you will need.[6]

The application process can be grueling, but it is probably one of the best things you can do for your child in the long run. You will need to collect a ton of information for the application, but keep in mind, you only have to do it one time and it's over.

If you are struggling with the application, you can always contact Family Voices, a nonprofit organization for promoting quality healthcare for children and youth. You can find them online at www.familyvoices.org or reach them toll free at 888-835-5669. They can give you helpful advice pertaining to SSI, but they can also help you find doctors and specialists in your area who take Medicaid.[7]

The downside to Medicaid is that not all doctors accept it because Medicaid pays less than insurance companies and may take months for reimbursement. It is unfortunate, but something we have to deal with. Another option is to contact Parent to Parent for help with the application process.

If your child is diagnosed with ASD but does not meet the criteria for the diagnostic code of 299.00 or F84.0, there is a chance they may still receive benefits through SSI. It is, however, very difficult to qualify without these particular diagnostic codes, which is really too bad. Kids with PDD or Asperger's need and deserve services, but it is not easy to get SSI with these diagnoses.

The autism spectrum is broad and, consequently, has many diagnostic (or medical) codes. If your child has Asperger's, Rett, or pervasive developmental disorder, the code will most likely be 299.80 (F84.5) but can be 299.00

(F84.0) if the doctor (or diagnosing professional) feels that the symptoms are severe enough to justify this code.

I have met many parents who have children with Asperger's, Rett, and PDD. What they go through trying to get services for their child is deplorable. Although high-functioning autism is less intense than classic autism, it is in no way easy or simple to treat. There is nothing easy or fun about being lonely or isolated, and many people with Asperger's struggle with socializing in a typical manner. High-functioning autism can be terribly hard on the person affected, and I hope that someday Medicaid and private insurance companies step up to the plate and start to address the needs of these individuals.

For now, however, it is tricky to qualify for benefits through SSI if your child is considered high-functioning. I encourage you to apply anyway and provide all of the information you can. Make copies of receipts you have for therapy, special diets, medication, etc. I would also encourage you to ask for written statements from your child's doctor pertaining to their *activities of daily living* (ADLs) and the support they need at home. Your child's doctor can also include any medical history and the need for therapy to ensure that age-appropriate social skills are taught by a trained behavioral therapist. Teachers, therapists, family, and friends can also provide statements. When you are applying for SSI, give them all of the information you can to justify the need for therapy. What I mean by that is *give them everything*: every piece of paper that is relevant to your child's medical/educational/social/emotional history. If you are denied, you always have the right to appeal, and I would recommend doing so. If your child has high-functioning autism, see the EPSDT section below.

There are many codes to indicate a child is on the autism spectrum. The website *ICD-10 Code Search* will give you a better understanding of what each diagnostic code means.[8] It outlines the various degrees of ASD and, again, can be beneficial when applying for Medicaid or justifying medical necessity to your private insurance company. No matter what the diagnostic code is, the fact remains the same—our kids need interventions and adequate care. When applying for Medicaid or approval from your insurance company, include the diagnostic code and every relevant therapy and intervention that may help the child become independent and self-sufficient. You are making the case that these interventions will save the insurance company money in the long run if they approve your application/claim. You aren't being dishonest or asking for something your child doesn't deserve. Do not feel bad about pleading your case or appealing the decision if denied SSI benefits.

Kids with high-functioning autism often need social-skills groups and vocational training (job or trade coaching) in order to succeed in their adult life. People with high-functioning autism can lead very lonely lives if they are not taught the social skills needed to form lasting relationships. Social skills are also vital for maintaining employment so that people with autism can work and make their own living. Such therapies and interventions for our kids will only benefit them and ultimately the taxpayers as they reach adulthood.

The purpose of SSI Medicaid, in my eyes, is to provide the necessary tools—via therapy and access to quality medical care—to ensure that the child will become a successful, independent adult (when possible). With the right support, a significant number of people with autism can thrive and live independently. But most importantly, they can be happy.

Each time you apply for any government program, including SSI, your application starts with the date you first applied. If their office "can't find" your application, you will have to start the application process over. If you take one piece of advice from me, please let it be this: *All correspondence must be mailed through the Post Office via certified mail.* It is critically important that you send *all* applications using certified mail; this ensures that there is a record of them having received your application and/or supporting documents. You can use the date on the receipt as the date of application. I can't tell you how many families I've worked with who didn't receive services because their applications were lost.

In general, the focus must always be on getting the child the best care available. Most of us, who cannot afford $30,000–50,000 per year in therapy, would need to apply for additional coverage, which brings me to my next point: applying for a Medicaid waiver or insurance-specific resources in your state.

MEDICAID WAIVERS

Each state is different when it comes to long-term care for a child with autism. For instance, the state I live in (Colorado) has ten Medicaid waivers, and David is only eligible for two of them. The word *waiver*, in this case, simply means that the parents' income requirement is waived, and parent(s) can make a decent living while their child receives Medicaid. If we did not have a waiver, I would have to stay under the income guidelines for SSI indefinitely.

In Colorado the waivers for children with disabilities include additional services such as behavioral therapy, summer camp for kids with autism, and respite care for the parent. As our children age, their waivers change, and they eventually transition to adult services. Waivers for adults include vocational coaching and living expenses. Unfortunately, adult waivers are very limited. The purpose of Medicaid waivers is to help the child reach their maximum potential by adulthood. Adult services, therefore, are minimal, making waivers best utilized by teaching the child functional, behavioral, and work-related skills before reaching the age of 18 or 21 depending on the waiver.

I know that the waiver program is new to many of you. In short, it is a program designed to support the functional and developmental needs of children with disabilities. The waiver does not count family income and may provide in-home care. They are often referred to as either the Katie Beckett or *Home & Community-Based Services* (HCBS) waivers. The waiver program was established in 1981 thanks to the tireless efforts of Katie Beckett's mother, Julie. The premise of the waiver program is that children are better cared for by their parents than a hospital or other institution.[9]

Many states that require insurance companies to cover autism-related services will specify a maximum benefit amount. The benefit amount could, for example, be $30,000 per year, which would be used to pay for a variety of services specifically intended for children with autism. This often includes behavior therapy, as social skills are something our children must be taught. These skills do not come naturally to children with autism but are a necessity if they are to work and be independent in adulthood.

Behavioral therapy encompasses a number of different therapies which can include *Applied Behavioral Analysis* (ABA), *Relationship Development Intervention* (RDI), or even after-school or summer programs, to name a few. Each state will specify the approved therapies and the dollar amount each family can spend.

The Medicaid waiver will cover therapy, not the little bit we can afford, but real therapy. In many cases, your child can receive ABA, RDI, speech, and occupational therapies under the waiver. Most waiver programs will require either a denial or approval letter from SSI, which is why I would apply for SSI before applying for a Medicaid waiver.

Keep in mind that the intention of the waiver is to get your child as healthy and as independent as possible before they reach adulthood. If the services provided by the waiver are used effectively, many people with autism will develop adequate vocational and social skills.

The kids who fully recover from autism generally have three things in common: (1) parents who are dedicated to their child's recovery, (2) biomedical interventions, and (3) therapy. Applying for the waiver is the first step in getting the therapy piece of the equation handled. Keep in mind, not all kids recover completely, but my son, for example, went from worst-case scenario for autism to high-functioning autism. There is always hope for a high quality of life for our kids, and the waiver can help achieve that goal.

I applied for the waiver when David was six and we didn't get it until he was 11, so it's imperative that you start the application process as soon as you can. We live in Colorado, and the last time I checked, we were 49th in funding for people with disabilities. We're one of the worst states in that regard, so keep faith. Odds are, your state will have more funding than we do, and you will not need to wait five years for services.

In Colorado a parent can apply for the Medicaid waiver through their community-centered board (CCB). Your CCB may be called something different. In California, for example, these organizations are called regional centers. Regardless of how they are named, these centers will help you locate and apply for available resources in your state. My CCB, for example, accepted my application and notified me when we had reached the top of the list.

Each state has these organizations which are typically funded through the department of human services and the developmental disabilities council for the state. These organizations will manage your child's budget for therapy and related services.

As I said earlier David did not get the waiver until a few years ago, and I feel that if he had gotten it at a younger age, he would have made more significant progress early on. Yes, he's doing well, but in the few years he's had the waiver, and therefore behavior therapy, he's made tremendous gains in both language and social skills.

If I had had the money I would have started these therapies years ago, but it just simply wasn't an option. The skills he's learned in the behavior therapy and social skills groups provided by the waiver are amazing. He's trying to make friends for the first time, he's playing board and interactive games with his peers, and his language has increased tremendously since he started behavior therapy. He's been saying funny things like, "Hey Aidan, how was school today?" And when Aidan was coughing at the dinner table, he said, "Stop being so dramatic, Aidan."

The therapists will work with you to determine appropriate goals for your child. David's goals always include aspects of safety awareness such as; safely crossing the street, what he's to do if he is separated from his family in public, and what to do in an emergency. We will continue to work on these skills every year until he has them down. As the parent you will help to determine which goals your child will work toward.

The effects of ABA, or whichever behavior therapy you choose, can be monumental in your child's development. These therapies are also very expensive, and the waitlist to receive services can be quite long in some states. In Colorado, in order to qualify for a waiver, a parent must provide a benefits approval or denial letter from Social Security, and the child must meet the criteria for the waiver. Therapies funded by the waiver can ultimately mean the difference between a child who can communicate and behave in a socially appropriate manner and one who cannot. It makes a huge difference to have these therapies covered by either a waiver or your insurance company.

In some instances, the waiver may also pay for respite care and, possibly, home modifications if they are deemed necessary in your child's service plan. There are websites which can help you to access information about waiver programs in your state; two are listed in the endnotes.[10] They may also be able to direct you to the CCB in your area. Once you've identified the CCB in your county, you can make an appointment with a resource coordinator. This person will do the initial screening, offer assistance with the waiver application process, and can direct you toward additional services in your county.

EPSDT

I met a man named Steven Kossor at the AutismOne Conference in Chicago a few years back. Kossor is a psychologist who started The Institute for Behavior Change in Pennsylvania.[11] His company develops treatment plans for children who have autism, ADHD, and other conditions. Steven has worked to develop treatment plans that are funded by EPSDT, which stands for *E*arly and *P*eriodic *S*creening, *D*iagnosis, and *T*reatment, the child health portion of Medicaid. He explains that, if your child has Medicaid, medical interventions and therapy are a civil right. His treatment plans are available on his website. Some can be accessed for free while other plans require a minimal fee. His company can help parents write a treatment plan that will fund behavior therapy and rehabilitative services. There is a consultation fee if you choose to go through the Institute for help with your treatment plan, but in the long run, it will save you money in out-of-pocket medical care for your child.[12]

The beauty of EPSDT funding is that your child does not have to qualify for SSI or a waiver to access medical care. EPSDT, under Medicaid, funds treatments that will "prevent disease, disability and other health conditions or their progression; prolong life; and promote physical and mental health and efficiency." Kossor's book, *The Issachar Project*, is available for purchase online if you would like to learn more about EPSDT and Medicaid.[13]

If your child has Medicaid, he/she qualifies for treatment under EPSDT until age 21. This funding source is incredibly important to families who do not qualify for SSI or a waiver. Accessing funding depends on writing an airtight treatment plan. Again, you can model your child's treatment plan based on the examples in Kossor's book or on his website. If you feel you'd benefit from consultation, it is definitely worth the money to have his company assist you in this process.

EPSDT funding can be a saving grace for children with high-functioning autism who have Medicaid. These kids need therapy and treatment to prepare for adulthood but are denied services on a regular basis. If your child is in this predicament, I highly recommend writing a treatment plan or reaching out to The Institute for Behavior Change for consultation.

AUTISM RESOURCES IN YOUR STATE

There are certain resources for people with autism available in every state. The first order of business is to establish the location of your disability resource center. When moms call me from other states, I want to provide them with this information, but unfortunately, it's difficult to find a national registry of these organizations.

The first problem is these agencies are called something different in every state. In Colorado, our disability resource center is called a *community-centered board*. In California, they are called *regional centers*. In Ohio, they are called *county boards of developmental disabilities*. Fun times. Anyway, these organizations are in every state and every county (large counties absorb smaller rural counties if necessary), and they receive (partial) funding from the federal government to ensure that people with disabilities can access local resources.

Disability resource centers can help parents find preschools for children with developmental disabilities, access state resources, apply for waivers, access recreational activities, vocational training, residential treatment, transportation, and family support. If you know your disability resource center, great. Give them a call and ask how to access services. If you don't know the name of this agency in your county, you can ask a school social worker. Call your school district's special education department, ask a pediatrician, call the Medicaid office in your state, or Google "department of developmental disabilities" in your state. I wish I could provide you with a simple list of these organizations, but unfortunately, I don't think one exists. Disability resource centers are also funded by states; therefore, each state oversees their budget and determines how funds are to be used. Accessing local resources is simplified by these agencies, which they can help streamline the process of.

You may also want to contact your local Autism Society chapter, Family Voices and/or Parent-to-Parent if you are struggling to find adequate health coverage and local resources for your child. These organizations should know which insurance options and specific resources are available in your state.

Another great resource, where available, is The Arc. They offer advocacy services (in some states) and help families access resources, recreational activities, and vocational and employment opportunities, and champion legislation for people with intellectual and developmental disabilities.[14] To find a chapter in your state or county, you can use the link provided at the end of the book.[15]

THE AFFORDABLE CARE ACT (ACA)

I am not an expert on the Affordable Care Act. Having said that, I do know that people, like our kids, who have a pre-existing condition can now access healthcare that would have previously been unavailable to them. In short, health insurance plans can't refuse to cover you or charge you more if you have a pre-existing health condition. The exception to this rule is individual health insurance plans, such as self-pay plans, not issued through an employer.

This means that if you don't have coverage, you now have the opportunity to apply for healthcare. I know that some of our kids do not qualify for SSI or Medicaid waivers but are denied coverage from insurance companies based on their pre-existing condition. The kids who are on the spectrum, do not have adequate health insurance, and who need therapy may benefit from the Affordable Care Act and the coverage provided by this legislation. Unfortunately, as you are probably aware, the current administration aims to revamp the ACA and continuation of these policies is in doubt, but as of this writing, they are still in place. You will need to select an insurance provider based on your needs. You can select from a variety of different plans, each with a different degree of coverage.

You'll want to select an insurance plan that has the highest number of therapy visits but be mindful of deductibles and co-pays. When my ex-husband was insuring David, we met the maximum out-of-pocket deductible rather quickly, which meant I no longer had to pay co-pays for visits after that point.

A good way to save money on healthcare is to track your expenses and make sure that, once you've reached the out-of-pocket maximum, you notify your insurance provider so they will cover the cost of care for the rest of the year, including co-pays. Once you have reached your out-of-pocket maximum, you should no longer receive bills for therapy or medical care.

States have their own agencies assigned to manage healthcare. You can call 1-800-318-2596 and get the phone number to your state's healthcare management office. Because each state is managing its own healthcare (even though it is federally funded), you will need to log onto your state's website in order to read about the plans that are available to you.

In the past when David was little and we lost our health insurance, we had no chance of him being covered without group insurance or Medicaid for his disability. It was a dismal time, and what's worse, millions of Americans with pre-existing conditions suffered the same fate.

As much as I wish the Affordable Care Act were simple and easy to understand, it is not. Not for me anyway. I will be the first to tell you that I do not know everything about the ACA or what it means for our kids. All I know for sure is that there are kids out there, right now, who have autism or a number of other health issues, who need help and because of the ACA they currently qualify for insurance. I'll take a complicated system over no coverage any day.

The ACA may not be as user-friendly as I'd like it to be, but at least you should be able to avoid the mountain of debt (and potential bankruptcy) that I accumulated during my marriage. I feel that it is truly unethical that millions of Americans suffered, and in some cases died, because they couldn't get insurance based on cost or a pre-existing condition. That is one thing I struggled with when David was at his worst. I felt that the country I love so dearly had become completely unethical in dealing with the poor and the sick. Up until then, I had never been either poor or sick. I had no idea that my children and I would be left defenseless. I always assumed that when people needed help, they got it.

At the end of the day, what matters most is your child with autism. Don't worry about people judging you if you have to use SSI or Children's Health Insurance Program (CHIP) in order to provide health insurance for your child. I mean, if they have an issue with it they can pay it, right? Right.

In my family I was the first person ever to accept any form of government help. I was embarrassed and ashamed, but there was literally no other option. I was on my own, and I had to make a lot of hard choices, that being one of them.

Looking back, when people made comments about David getting SSI, I wish I had handled it differently. I was so defeated and heartbroken that I could barely manage what was on my plate, let alone defend myself.

If someone tried to make me feel guilty now, my response would be something like this, "I worked and went to school from the ages of fifteen to twenty-three, and the only reason I stayed home after David was born was because he was too sick for me to work. I would gladly work eighty hours a week if it meant he could have his childhood back. I would trade in his handicapped parking placard and park in the last spot of every parking lot for the rest of my natural life if it meant he would be healthy."

The difference between the way I handle things now and how I handled them before is like night and day. I took it all to heart back then, but I learned some valuable lessons along the way. Most people wouldn't last a day in our shoes, so why would we listen to their criticism? I hear people in stores complaining about the temperature not being right, or they were overcharged a dollar on their bill. All I can think is, *You think that's a real problem?*

Having a child with health issues, now *that* is a real problem. Having to choose between medical bills and groceries, that is a real problem. The thing about David having autism, allergies, sensory issues, and asthma is that I know what a real problem is. Everything else seems trivial.

If what they say is true, "what doesn't kill you makes you stronger," most of us will come out of this like warriors— you know, like Spartan 300-type warriors. When you've been through as much as we have, you don't have to take crap from anyone.

Be a warrior about things. Don't let people make you feel bad; there is no shame in doing what is right for your child. Right now you are planting the seeds for a fruitful and healthful adulthood for your child. If people judge you, hand them your child's medical bills and politely say, "You are welcome to pay these if you'd like. If not, there's the door."

I realize that we, as parents, have to make a lot of hard decisions. Decisions we'd rather not have to make. In the end, regardless of which insurance you have, be it private or group insurance, Medicaid/social security, or a policy under the ACA, the objective remains the same. Your child needs health insurance in order to lead a happy and (hopefully) independent life as an adult.

Yes, this will take, time, energy, a ton of patience. In your quest for finding the right coverage remember to weigh your options and find the plan that best meets the needs of your family.

Each person with autism has different needs, but they all need health insurance. Trust yourself and your ability to make the right decision in terms of selecting the right type of insurance plan. If you have existing insurance and do not need to make any changes, that's great! If not, the road ahead looks a lot worse than it really is. Just keep your eye on the prize, and it will all come together.

The initial paperwork for any type of new insurance is awful, but just remember, you only do it once and it's over. Starting with a new insurance plan or applying for Medicaid benefits is the metaphoric equivalent to "planting seeds": You won't have a harvest tomorrow, but your child will in 20 years. Remember that when you want to throw the application (or your computer) out the window when applying for benefits!

Never give up!

NOTES FOR CHAPTER 3

4

BIOMEDICAL INTERVENTIONS FOR AUTISM: RECOVERY IS POSSIBLE

My doctors told me I would never walk again. My mother told me I would. I believed my mother.

—Wilma Rudolph

I KNOW, I KNOW, we're often told by our doctors that "there is no cure," "your child may never live independently," or "he will never speak." However, there are many parents and organizations that will not agree with these dismal prognoses. In fact, there are countless stories of children who have completely recovered from autism.

There is no better time for recovery than now, so let's get to it! Here's the list of topics I'll touch on to help you recover your child:

- Biomedical interventions
- Then and now, stories of recovery
- Embracing a changing lifestyle
- Things you should know before you vaccinate

BIOMEDICAL INTERVENTIONS

Biomedical interventions focus on the biological needs of the individual and not the umbrella diagnosis of autism. Sidney Baker explains it best in *Autism: Effective Biomedical Treatments*: "Even in the midst of an epidemic in which we assume the victims 'have the same thing,' respect for each person's differences is the key to finding that person's best diagnostic and therapeutic options."[1]

Baker elaborates and explains how it all started, "In 1995, 32 clinicians, researchers and parents gathered to form a consensus concerning the most scientifically credible biomedical diagnostic and treatment choices available to children on the autism spectrum." He goes on to say, "Even though some children have become cured as a result of simple interventions, none of us whose opinions form the basis of this book believes that the answers to this puzzle are, or will soon be, simple."[2]

There are no simple answers to the question of what is causing the exponential rise in autism rates. There is, however, plenty of information on how to treat it successfully. For me, the hardest things about getting the diagnosis for David were that I didn't know what questions to ask, how to treat his symptoms, or even where to start.

Although there are no "simple" answers, there are solutions. Our kids can get better, though let me be the first to tell you, it's going to take time, dedication, and heart. Biomedical interventions include a variety of treatments, and some of them are time consuming and costly. However, nothing is more time consuming than a child with autism who is struggling with negative behaviors. And nothing can compare financially to the cost of caring for a child for the rest of his or her life.

The time and money that goes into biomedical treatments is nothing compared to the total cost of long-term care for a person with severe autism. The stress of changing

David's diet was minimal in contrast to the stress I felt when he had cataclysmic meltdowns. I say this because I don't want you to read this chapter and think you have yet one more thing to add to your busy schedule. In fact, based on my own experience, the opposite is true; these interventions have freed me up financially and emotionally, and my stress level is the lowest it's been since the onset of his symptoms.

When I first read about biomedical interventions, I was at the end of my rope. I was stressed beyond belief, and around that time, I remember feeling as if I wouldn't be able to manage much longer. One day, I was driving home from work and David was having a *really* bad day.

At the time he could not tolerate any deviations in our routine. When I picked him up from day care, he started screaming (something he did almost every car ride) and proceeded to scream and kick throughout the 45-minute drive home. Because he needed a predictable routine, I drove the same exact way home every day after work. This day, however, there was a car accident and I was forced to take an unfamiliar route home.

This small change in routine pushed David over the edge. He started kicking so hard, I thought he was going to break the back window. He did break off the door lock and was spitting at me and his brother. I knew that if I pulled the car over it would only make him worse, so I kept driving, gripping the steering wheel so tightly my knuckles were pure white. Poor Aidan was in the backseat with David reaching for him, trying to scratch and kick him. I felt like I was being torn in half. I love both kids so much, and I felt at that moment that I wasn't able to protect either one of them—a hollow feeling for a mother. The screaming and kicking was terrifying. At the time, David was four and Aidan was two, and I just couldn't see me being able to raise them under these circumstances until their eighteenth birthdays.

There was only one day care that would take David, and it meant that I had to drive 45 minutes there and then another 45 minutes to work. I drove three hours a day, every day I worked. If there was traffic or a snowstorm, it was closer to a four-hour drive per day. The combination of my crazy driving schedule, having no husband, no money, no breaks, and no hope of things changing pushed me to my limits. In addition to the stress I felt, I had a sinking feeling that abuse was occurring at the day care, but when you have no one to rely on, what do you do? *Do I quit my job to stay home with him? How will I buy food, gas, clothes, etc.?* It was a seemingly hopeless situation. On top of that when I called Social Services to see if they could send someone out to check the day care, they said that they couldn't if the child could not testify. Great.

On this particular day, with David screaming bloody murder for 40 minutes straight, I lost it. As I drove I cried out at the top of my lungs, "God, why are you doing this? I can't take another day.... Please have mercy.... Please have mercy, God. Please have mercy on us!" I must have said, "Please have mercy on us" about a hundred more times on our drive home. I didn't know what else to do; I had no answers, and all rational thought had been drowned out by the screams of my son. I was broken, and the only hope of me being whole again was directly linked to God's grace and my son's health. The two would go hand-in-hand as I would soon find out.

Shortly after this terrible day, David's therapist handed me the article (as mentioned in chapter 2), "Daniel's Success Story: A Determined Mother Demonstrates that Full Recovery from Autism Is Possible," by Mary Romaniec. I read it and felt the only peace I had felt in four years. I knew then that God had heard my cries for mercy. He saw that I needed hope to move on, and that's exactly what that article gave me. Hope.

When I read the article, I noticed that the author's son's symptoms were very similar to David's. I don't mean the symptoms of autism; I mean the physical symptoms that would necessitate biomedical interventions.

The author's son, Daniel, "had terrible green diarrhea." Daniel's language, like David's, decreased and soon became nothing but a memory. David spoke a few words, knew his alphabet and some numbers at 13 months, but soon after, regressed and stopped speaking entirely. Daniel, like David, would often be found "banging his head against the wall and writhing on the ground." As I read about this little boy, I felt a sense of sadness for him and his family, but I also felt a sense of belonging; I was not in this alone. I knew that if one mother could get her son better, I could get mine better too. And so it began.

Her article recommended books and resources to start the journey toward recovery. She suggested that readers look into ARI (Autism Research Institute), which I did, and boy, did it change everything.

I was ready to get started on our road to recovery, and I didn't want to wait for the book from ARI to come in the mail. I printed out a chart from ARI that lists the biomedical interventions commonly used for children with autism and started our journey to recovery that day.

The chart outlines the efficacy of various interventions. Some of the interventions listed are prescription drugs, and I chose not to give David these medications. Instead, I opted for the "Biomedical and Non-drug Supplements."[3]

After reading up on each intervention, I felt they were safe and would garner fewer side effects than prescription drugs. I chose the most effective biomedical interventions on the list and promised myself I would follow through with each one. By the time I read the chart, David had already been tested for food allergies, so I had already removed oat, peanut, soy, rice, and gluten from his diet. Shortly after that, I also removed casein (a protein found in dairy products).

I went to ARI's website and found it to be incredibly helpful. I immediately ordered the book, *Autism: Biomedical*

Interventions and started researching our options. I always kept "Daniel's Story" in the back of my mind and close to my heart as I read the book from ARI. When I would start to lose hope that David could improve, I would read the article again for inspiration. The part of Mary's article that really hooked me was this line, "Our son went from two words in January of 2002 to full sentences by July 2002."

I realized then that, with the help of ARI and this mother's advice, I too could get my son speaking or, at a minimum, I could get him to stop the incessant screaming, hitting, and kicking. I am skeptical of most things, so I really did my homework. I read article after article about biomedical interventions, and I read countless stories of children who had recovered completely.

Dietary Interventions

Removing gluten, casein, and soy were monumental in David's development. He began looking at me, he stopped hitting and kicking, and he was signing a couple words. In essence, he was a different child. I attribute his drastic behavioral changes to simply feeling better. The food allergies he had (unbeknownst to me) were surely causing him headaches and tummy aches, and the gluten and casein were inflaming his digestive tract, resulting in chronic diarrhea. Who wouldn't be grumpy if they had a headache and diarrhea every day?

I think that it's worth trying the gluten-free/casein-free/soy-free (GF/CF/SF) diet to see if your child responds positively. When it comes to the diet, I've heard it all. Many parents are reluctant to try the diet. I've heard "It's too hard," "It's too expensive," and/or "He's a picky eater," more times than I can count. These things are true for most of our kids. But I promise you this, if the diet works for your child, and they start to improve, you will not regret a single day or even a moment you spent researching and preparing foods.

The diet costs a little bit more, but again, what is the cost of caring for our kids for the rest of their lives? Starting the diet wasn't a fun transition, don't get me wrong. David loves blueberry muffins, milk, and crackers and taking these things away wasn't easy. He had major meltdowns, and we matched wits for a month or so. The bottom line is this: I'm the adult, I buy the food, I decide what he eats. Sorry, Charlie.

There are sound reasons for trying the diet, and in all honesty, I've heard nothing but good things from parents who stick to it. Many parents have told me that they tried the diet and "it didn't work." When I probed further, it turned out these parents had been sending their children to school where the children were eating school lunch. If a child is eating school lunch or eats what they want at Grandma's house, they are not eating gluten-free, casein-free, or soy-free. I've never met anyone who followed through with the diet and didn't see major improvements. The half-hearted approach does not work. You'll need to be "all in" to see results. Keep in mind, there are a variety of diets we can try. Some parents try the Specific Carbohydrate (SCD) or the GAPS (Gut and Psychology Syndrome) diets if the GF/CF/SF diet isn't effective.

The diet requires total commitment; everything your child eats must be approved by you. It's a tough transition at first, but David has been on the diet for eleven years now, and it's an integrated part of our lives. It's really no big deal once you're used to it. As a volunteer Mentor for Talk about Curing Autism (TACA), I know TACA has exceptional resources and advice on the diet. Their website has recipe ideas, shopping tips, meal plans, and more. It's a great resource for parents who are just getting started. TACA's website states:

> Be committed. Know that research shows that 91% of ASD kids improve on the GFCFSF diet. The diet will only make your child healthier, and healthy is

the goal after all. Yes, the diet can be confusing at first, but everything you will need is on the TACA website. And remember this, YOU CAN DO IT!!![4]

The scientific explanation of the diet is very complicated. It comes down to proteins and the body's inability to break them down and digest them properly. The undigested proteins can essentially leak into the blood and are then carried to the brain. Another key point is that, if your child is having chronic diarrhea or constipation, they most certainly have an inflamed digestive tract; 80-90% of neurotransmitters—the chemicals our bodies use to transmit signals from neuron to neuron—are made in the gut, and this is also where serotonin, an important chemical in "happiness," is produced. If the gut is inflamed due to food intolerance, there will be neurological symptoms and the child's mood will be unpredictable based on the disrupted production of serotonin. The immune system is linked to the gut as well, so it's important to address gastrointestinal issues (GI) as soon as possible.

I'm a mom, and as a mom I know that the last thing you need is more medical jargon. I would strongly recommend, however, that you look into the science behind the diet. You would be well served to research the diet and come to your own conclusions. It's a big commitment, but the reward can be a happy and healthy child. It's worth the investment of time, energy, and money.

The diet is a huge transition, did I mention that enough times? I don't want you to struggle, and I know that finding foods our kids will eat can be challenging. Meals become easier when you make something everyone can eat. Sometimes it may just be the main course but coming up with foods everyone enjoys will save you time in the kitchen. Below are a few meal and snacking ideas which may help your child acclimate quickly:

Fruits and veggies: Most of our kids won't eat them, but if yours does, count your lucky stars and try to make plant-based meals. Try to buy organic as often as possible.

Whole chicken: I buy (organic) whole chickens and rub them with olive oil, salt, and garlic. It's simple, and everyone loves it!

Chicken wings: I use olive oil, salt, and gluten-free organic barbeque sauce.

Chicken sandwiches: Use whatever chicken your family likes (as long as it isn't pre-flavored) and add Daiya or another dairy-free cheese to your child's sandwich. It's tricky to get the dairy-free cheese to melt, so I put oil in the pan, put the sandwich together, and put something heavy on top of it to help the cheese melt.

Bacon cheese fries: I buy organic French fries; add a little salt, Daiya dairy-free cheese, and bacon pieces.

Grilled cheese: We have tried several gluten-free breads. In my opinion, the best-tasting option is Canyon House gluten/casein-free. I use Canyon House bread with the Daiya pepper jack cheese, and David loves it. I recommend making the gluten-free sandwich first or separately from the other grilled cheese sandwiches because cross-contamination can be an issue. David has his own toaster, and I cook his food separately from ours, so it isn't "contaminated" by gluten from our bread.

Meatballs: Most health food stores, or online food stores, carry GF/CF/SF breadcrumbs for meatballs. David does not like the texture of onion or garlic, so I grind them up in the food processor before adding them to the mixture.

Bob's Red Mill: Their GF/CF/SF cake mixes have a good flavor. I make David the cookies, too, but

add a little organic vanilla and dairy-free choco-
late to the mix.

Udi's: It is very important for our kids to eat organic
foods as often as possible. Udi's is not organic,
but if you are just getting started, you'll want to
make the transition as painless as possible. Their
muffins are delicious and don't taste much different from what kids are used to eating.

Applegate: Applegate makes tasty GF/CF/SF
chicken nuggets and chicken strips and has a
variety of organic lunchmeats to choose from.

Surf Sweets: This brand makes organic GF jelly
beans, gummy bears, and fruit snacks.

Clif Kid: They have fruit ropes for snacks that are all
organic and made with real fruit and veggies.

Stretch Island fruit leather: This is a great healthy
alternative to conventional fruit leather.

Cheesecake: Daiya makes different types of cheese-
cakes. I buy them on holidays or if we are going
to a birthday party. I want David to have the same
foods, including desserts, everyone else is eating.
It's an easy way to address desserts at parties
and holiday functions.

Mac and cheese: Daiya makes a GF/CF/SF mac
and cheese. However, your child may need to
adjust to the diet before taking to this brand's
version of mac and cheese. It does not taste like
conventional versions and takes some getting
used to.

French toast: David can eat everything we eat for
breakfast with a few simple modifications. I make
his french toast with goat's milk, organic vanilla,
a little brown sugar, and egg. I fry everything in
olive oil and he loves it!

Donuts: Kinnikinnick makes different flavors of
donuts that are GF/CF/SF.

Chips: David eats Boulder brand chips, and occasionally he'll eat Tostitos brand organic corn chips. Both brands are tasty and don't have a ton of preservatives and artificial flavoring.

Breakfast sandwiches: Most of our kids have sensory issues and oral sensitivity can create issues around food. David used to eat his foods separately, and the separate foods were never allowed to touch. As the oral sensitivity has decreased, he now eats a variety of foods, including combinations like breakfast sandwiches. If your child tends to gag or is not comfortable mixing foods, there is no need to rush. Sensory issues typically improve with biomedical interventions, occupational therapy, or feeding therapy and will decrease over time. That being said, if your child will tolerate mixing foods, you can make breakfast sandwiches with GF/CS/SF bread, bacon or sausage, eggs, and dairy-free cheese.

Drinks: Santa Cruz makes a variety of lemonades. Honest Kids has great juices for school lunches, and Hansen's has an organic juice box option for school lunches as well. Organic juice contains real fruit juice and does not have artificial flavors or food dyes. In your quest to go GF/CF/SF, you will want to consider adding organic foods and drinks with the fewest artificial ingredients.

This is a short list of foods to get you started on the diet. You will find foods your child likes as time goes by. Dietary changes are a marathon, not a sprint. You will find a rhythm with meal and snack times, but it doesn't all have to happen overnight. Be easy on yourself during this time; it's a tough transition, and your child will probably go through symptoms of what look like withdrawal from gluten. They will throw tantrums, behaviors may increase for a month or so, and they will most likely resist these changes. Hold your ground and tough it out. The diet is a necessary piece of recovery. When you want to quit, visualize your child being happy. Visualize your child communicating and doing well in school. Your child can recover or greatly improve. Stick to it and remember the battle cry of autism parents around the world: **Never give up**!

Detox

Moving down the list the next biomedical intervention I chose was detox. What ARI means by detox in this context is chelation. Chelation is, in a nutshell, the process of removing heavy metals from the body. All people have small amounts of heavy metals in their bodies. The difference is that our kids tend to have extraordinarily high levels of heavy metals in their little bodies. The best analogy for heavy-metal toxicity is the Mad Hatter character we've come to know from *Alice in Wonderland*. Mad hatter disease is a real thing, not just a quirky fictional reference. It was caused by mercury exposure and reached its peak in the early 1800s when milliners (hat makers) used mercury-based solutions in the production and formation of hats. Millineries were often poorly ventilated, and many hat makers fell ill and developed what is now known as mad hatter disease. People with mad hatter disease may have tremors, diarrhea, sensory processing issues, neurological dysfunction (ataxia), and may become socially withdrawn. The symptoms of mad hatter disease are essentially those of mercury poisoning. These symptoms are strikingly similar to the symptoms of autism. The purpose of testing for heavy metals and chelating a child who has a high toxic body burden is to address and eventually reverse the symptoms of mercury exposure and/or heavy-metal toxicity.

I believe the most effective method of testing for heavy metals is with a provocation agent. You must first provoke the metals with a chelating agent, typically DMSA or DMPS (different versions of chelators). Parents give their child DMSA (for example) for a trial period and test either their urine or stool for heavy-metal toxicity. Unprovoked hair or urine tests for heavy-metal toxicity are a crap shoot. I tried testing David's hair, and the results were negative because most heavy metals can only be detected in hair immediately following exposure. When I tested for heavy-metal toxicity with the provocation agent DMSA, I learned that the heavy metal levels in David's body were high enough to shut down his liver and kidneys. David didn't just have heavy-metal toxicity, he had heavy-metal poisoning.

When I tested David, I wasn't expecting the results we got. I thought that he might have had metals in his body, but I never dreamed that it was so severe. His heavy-metal toxicity report is scary to look at, even today. How did those metals get into my four-year-old's body? Had I not read Mary Romaniec's article, I would not have tested my son using a chelator and David probably would not be with us today.

When I look back I can't even count the number of specialists I took him to and not one of them suspected heavy-metal toxicity. In the autism world I've come to learn other parents are often the best resource. In our case, Mary Romaniec saved my son's life. Because of her, he is now happier and more social than I was told would be possible. Recovering your child requires that you access varied sources of information. Unfortunately, most pediatricians receive very limited autism education in school. It's up to us to find answers and work with our pediatricians toward recovery. David's doctors all thought I was nuts when I put him on the diet and started detox, but he has made such remarkable progress that they now congratulate me and tell me what a great job I've done.

Although chelation is the most common form of heavy-metal detox, there are also other avenues to pursue. A couple years ago a friend of mine suggested I put David in a study for the IonCleanse by A Major Difference (AMD) detox footbath sponsored by Thinking Moms' Revolution. David had hit a plateau and was not making gains. I put him in the study because, to be honest, I didn't know what else to do. I'd done just about everything I could think of, and he simply wasn't getting better. He wasn't regressing, but he certainly wasn't developing new skills either. We had hit a wall.

I put him in the study thinking it would be another letdown, and yet I have never been more wrong. After four months of using the IonCleanse, his ATEC score dropped from 29 to 11, ATEC is the Autism Treatment Evaluation Checklist used to monitor the effectiveness of any given therapy or intervention.[5] He was making better eye contact, his language was increasing every week, he was more focused, and he even started making witty jokes on a regular basis. It changed everything for him. Once the study concluded, I bought an IonCleanse for our house, and as we continue to detox, he continues to improve.

I tried to grasp the science behind the IonCleanse, but it was a little over my head. I did learn, however, that it essentially opens up the detox pathways and allows the body to rid itself of toxins. Many of our children cannot methylate properly. If the methylation process is disrupted, the body can't detox efficiently. Because so many of our children have issues with methylation, it makes sense that they respond so well to the IonCleanse. They need to clear out the toxic body burden to heal the symptoms that present themselves as autism.

What's interesting about the IonCleanse is that the older the child is, the better they seem to respond. People say there is a window for recovery from autism, and until we tried the IonCleanse, I believed that. Now I think just about anyone with autism, regardless of age, can make significant gains with this method of detox. If our children can't detox adequately on their own, it makes perfect sense this method would help decrease the autism-like symptoms.

Some parents detox heavy metals naturally using things like cilantro, chlorella, and garlic. Dr. Dietrich Klinghardt has his own protocol that many parents find helpful.[6] Another woman I met used modified citrus pectin to address her heavy-metal toxicity.

Another alternative to traditional chelation is the Andy Cutler method of low-and-slow chelation. It's a gradual process, but the parents who try it seem to be happy with the results.[7] In our case David's heavy-metal poisoning was about to shut down his liver and kidneys according to his doctor, so I didn't have the option of gradual or natural methods of chelation. We started chelation using DMSA that day. The doctor said it was the worst heavy-metal toxicity report he'd ever seen and that David's liver and kidneys probably wouldn't last another week without chelation. Not all children will be in an emergency situation like David was. If your child's heavy-metal toxicity report shows low-level toxicity, you can always try the Andy Cutler protocol or a natural approach.

It's important to consult with an expert on chelation. I had a MAPS doctor advising me on how to approach detox and how to build David's body back up from the damage. In my experience, chiropractors seem to know quite a bit about natural healing. I always thought they focused primarily on adjustments and musculoskeletal issues, but it turns out I was wrong about that, too (dang it). Chiropractors actually have as many, if not more, education hours in anatomy and physiology, diagnosis, dermatology, ears, eyes, nose, throat, neurology, x-ray, and orthopedics than medical doctors.[8] They are highly qualified physicians who may be able to help your child if regular pediatricians are not able to identify and address underlying medical conditions. In some cases, like mine, all of the child's doctors are valued and offer advice. Sometimes, it can take more than one doctor to get to the root of the problem(s).

If you are considering detox, finding the right physician is key. That may be an alternative medicine doctor or a MAPS doctor.[9] Detox is key to recovery; a child cannot and will not recover from autism if they have high levels of heavy metals in their body. Heavy metals bind themselves intracellularly (they are hidden inside cells) and will wreak havoc on the body until they are removed. It is generally an essential part of recovery, and you, as a parent, will have to determine which chelation approach is best for your child. Find a good doctor who knows how to treat children with autism or, at a minimum, how to safely address chelation.

Digestive enzymes

In the early stages of the diet, David had some major food infractions. He would either sneak food or a sympathetic family member would feed him something he wasn't supposed to have. In these instances, I would give him digestive enzymes to help break down the proteins in the food he'd eaten.

I buy digestive enzymes for children at my local health food store. They are relatively inexpensive and help decrease the severity of his body's reaction to eating gluten or casein. If David ate gluten, for example, he'd get dark circles under his eyes, his eczema would return, and his poop would be runny. I always knew when he'd gotten into the wrong types of food and would give him enzymes as soon as I spotted the physical symptoms of a food infraction. While it helped decrease the severity of the reaction to these foods, it was not a replacement for the diet.

A few years into the diet, my mom bought a book called *Enzymes for Autism and Other Neurological Conditions* by Karen DeFelice.[10] This book gives very thorough and logical reasons as to why our kids benefit from enzymes. The book also recommends buying digestive enzymes formulated for kids with autism from Houston Enzymes. I bought AFP Peptizide and Zyme Prime for years from this company. David no longer needs enzymes, but in the thick of things,

Houston Enzymes were a saving grace for him; they meant the difference between a full regression into autism and a minor skin rash.

Methyl B12

I chose methyl B12 as an intervention simply because it was listed on the chart as an effective biomedical treatment for autism. I did a ton of research on it before I committed to giving it to David, but in the end, I feel it was probably one of the best things I could have done for him.

If I were writing a book on biomedical interventions, I would get into methylation more, but because I'm trying to keep this short and to the point, I'll just cover the basics. Methylation is a process in the body that is responsible for our stress response (fight or flight), glutathione production, detoxification of heavy metals, repairing cellular damage, genetic expression of DNA, energy, and immune cell production. In short, methylation is a vital part of detox and the maintenance of good health. If the methylation process is hindered, the body will never fully heal.

The reason that I, and countless other parents of children with autism, have chosen to use methyl B12 as an intervention is to help our kids detox on their own. I gave David methyl B12 subcutaneously off and on for several years. I gave it to him in injections every three days and asked his MAPS doctor to prescribe glutathione cream to aid in detoxification.

Methyl B12 injections (you can use a prescription lotion if your child won't tolerate shots) help repair damage done to the methylation process. About 90% of kids with autism have impaired methylation and can't detox on their own efficiently. Methyl B12 helps kick-start the methylation process, and the body will slowly start to detox. The brain is dependent upon B12, and what I saw in David after a few months on the shots was better eye contact, more awareness of his surroundings, and improved behaviors including the ability to meaningfully participate during therapy and at school.

It is a common intervention in our community simply because most of our kids can't detox effectively on their own. It helps their little bodies get rid of environmental toxins and should improve symptoms after a few months. If you choose to pursue this biomedical treatment option, I'd recommend talking to your physician about adding glutathione cream to help speed up the detox process.

On a side note, understanding methylation is critical to recovery. Since our children typically can't methylate properly, they have high toxicity levels. Dr. Amy Yasko has a really insightful book that can help you understand recovery and methylation if you are interested. As of this writing, it is free online.[11] Dr. Yasko also explains the need for genetic testing for kids with autism. My son has a methylenetetrahydrofolate reductase (MTHFR) genetic mutation we caught in his genetic testing. This mutation can spell disaster for children who are exposed to toxins because they cannot excrete them efficiently. Her book explains the role of MTHFR in regard to detoxification and the role of the immune system, which genetic tests to run, gut health, diet and supplements. It's truly a valuable resource for parents, and it's FREE!

Parasites

Over the course of ten years, I included every biomedical intervention I could from ARI chart. Although David improved and was doing great, he was still not recovered. Fast forward to a couple years ago, his health took a nose dive. He had terrible dark circles again under his eyes again, chronic headaches, and he was vomiting once or twice a week (which he didn't tell me about until it had been happening for two months). He was unable to get up in the morning for school, and he wasn't speaking much. It was heartbreaking to see him in that condition. I took him to his pediatrician who said David may be having migraine headaches which often start in puberty; he recommended giving him magnesium as a supplement. Magnesium helped with the headaches—he was no longer complaining of his head "feeling like Donkey Kong smash my head"—but he was still very lethargic and continued to have a hard time getting out of bed in the morning.

I took him to another pediatrician who sent us for blood work which came back normal. Then we went to the allergy doctor who didn't have any answers either. We did more blood work; what came up were viral issues.

I ended up taking him to a nutritionist who thought he may have parasites. She recommended supplements to address parasites and, within a couple months, he was on the mend. Again, doctors were only able to help minimally when he got sick. David has very good doctors but because medical school does not emphasize the principles of biomedical interventions and addressing environmental toxicity in children, many pediatricians miss these symptoms. Sometimes, other professionals need to be included, even with the care of a good doctor.

The nutritionist who saw David explained that because many children with autism have suppressed immune systems, it can lead to gut disturbances, including low stomach acid. She said food allergies cause additional stress on the gut and can lead to high-level parasitic infection deep within the tissues of the body. There are about 300 types of parasites that can use humans as a host, and our kids have the perfect storm of gut issues and compromised immune systems to allow parasites to flourish. The nutritionist recommended a supplement to get rid of the parasites gradually and, as parasites feed off sugar, told me to cut out sugar as much as possible.

After a few months of treating parasites, David was back to his old self. He was getting out of bed easily in the morning, his language returned, he was focused in school again, and was back to being my happy little guy.

Vitamins and supplements

David has taken more vitamins and supplements than I can recall. He needed vitamins for deficiencies we discovered through his blood work and supplements to address a number of issues. Our kids are all different and benefit from different vitamins and supplements based on their lab results. If you see a regular pediatrician, you can ask for blood work to check for vitamin deficiencies. If you see a holistic practitioner, they may do a muscle test instead of blood work. A MAPS doctor will most likely order blood, stool, and urine tests to determine whether your child is deficient in certain vitamins and would benefit from supplementation.

I have many friends who have kids with autism, and none of our kids take the exact same things; I will list a few examples of the things David takes to give you an idea of how these interventions work and why we give our kids vitamins and supplements to improve their health.

David takes **magnesium** to help with chronic headaches, but magnesium can be used to help decrease symptoms of anxiety, muscle spasms and sleep disturbances as well.[12] He also takes vitamins C and D3 to boost his immune system. He takes probiotics (recommended by his MAPS doctor) to maintain gut health, and manuka honey occasionally as it is a natural antiviral.

Just as other biomedical interventions are intended to address the unique needs of the individual child, vitamins and supplements will be specific to their needs as well. There is no one-size-fits-all approach. Our best bet is to consult with a healthcare professional to determine which vitamins and supplements will benefit our child the most.

Hyperbaric oxygen therapy

My decision to try hyperbaric oxygen therapy (HBOT) was based on the ARI Chart for Biomedical Interventions and the positive feedback I'd heard about it from other parents. One autism mom said her child was speaking more and had stopped perseverating (repeating words, phrases, or actions) after a few months of HBOT. Over the years I've met several parents who have used HBOT to treat their child's autism or physical disabilities; most parents report notable gains in fine and gross motor skills as well as increased communication. Unfortunately, David would not sit through the treatments, and I was not able to pursue this as an intervention for him. On a side note, it is important to mention that there is some debate on whether or not HBOT is a good option if a child has parasites. This is something you will want to research and speak to a healthcare professional about before committing to this particular intervention.

TACA has thorough explanations of many biomedical interventions on their website. For HBOT it says:

Some doctors are still studying the effects of HBOT treatment for children affected with autism to see if it helps treating co-morbid issues. Issues could include:

healing the gut and brain inflammation (two that
    may be separate issues or experienced
    simultaneously)
blood flow to key areas of the brain
dealing with gut parasites, yeast or bacteria
help in all four areas[13]

Candida

Candida is a fungus, a form of yeast that lives in the mouth and intestinal tract. When candida overgrowth occurs, it can break down the intestinal walls and contribute to leaky gut. Candida overgrowth can occur for a number of reasons. In David's case, I believe the excessive use of anti-biotics to treat constant ear and sinus infections until age five created a bacterial imbalance in his gut. The candida overgrowth most likely contributed to his skin rashes and diarrhea. His doctor detected candida overgrowth through a stool test. He recommended I treat the candida by decreasing his sugar intake and giving him probiotics. After a few months of the GF/CF/SF diet, probiotics and decreased sugar intake, his skin rashes cleared up and his poo was a bit more formed.

Warning: When your child is going through yeast die-off, they will be mad for about thirty days. Activated charcoal or Alka-Seltzer Gold will help absorb the bacterial and yeast die-off that triggers behavior. Yeast die-off is very difficult on the child but is necessary for gut health. There will most likely be increased behaviors and probably some loud vocalizations. A good pair of headphones for mom and dad and a solid playlist of your favorite songs will be a necessary tool in your surviving the yeast die-off.

What now?

I have done everything on the list from ARI I could do. A few years ago, David hit a plateau. He wasn't regressing, but he wasn't making gains either. It was so frustrating because I know there are parents who did half of what I did, and their children are no longer on the spectrum. I have always maintained the belief that David can and will recover, despite the severity of his autism; it is just a matter of discovering which underlying medical condition has not yet been addressed. As I mentioned, he improved dramatically after I gave him supplements to rid his body of parasites. Although treating parasites was enormously beneficial to his health, I knew I was still missing a piece to the recovery puzzle. Again, a friend suggested I put David in a study for The IonCleanse by (AMD). A previous study, also sponsored by Thinking Moms' Revolution, showed very promising results for our kids. The particular study we were in was specifically for teenagers who had autism. The study data below demonstrates a significant decrease in the symptoms of autism.41 The point is when you think you've done everything you can to recover your child, don't lose hope. Ask yourself, what now? What else can I do to help my child make gains? I live by the saying, "Where there is a will there is a way." There is always a way. Never give up!

The IonCleanse by AMD

The IonCleanse was a lifesaver for us. I can't even put into words how well David is doing since we started this protocol. He's not the same kid he was before the IonCleanse. He's doing better than ever, he's happier than he's ever been, he's socializing (in his own way), and is trying to start conversations. David is not the exception to the rule. Teenagers with autism are responding incredibly well to the IonCleanse. Below are the observations of the study data: 27 of 27 kids in the study had marked reductions in their ATEC scores.[14] It can be a game changer for some of our kids. Keep in mind every person's body responds differently to biomedical interventions. Although David responded well to the IonCleanse, I have heard of kids having increased autistic behaviors after starting the protocol, but the behaviors eventually decreased as the toxic body burden was lessened. Another child was doing the IonCleanse for six months, and her water never showed anything significant. One day she dumped so many metals, they thought the machine had broken into pieces, but it hadn't. Her body retained heavy metals like a magnet apparently, then one day, the detox pathways opened up and she was able to finally rid her body of the toxic burden. Like all interventions, it may take time before you see results, but the payoff is worth the wait. The only downside to the IonCleanse is that it can deplete minerals. It is suggested that parents supplement with trace minerals as a precaution. The cleanse can also rid the body of medications. If a person is taking anti-seizure medication, for example, the IonCleanse could potentially rid the body of needed anticonvulsants. In the case of children who take medication for seizures, this is probably not your best option.

The study showed very promising results for kids with autism. If this is something you'd like to try, you can contact AMD for more information.[15]

OBSERVATIONS:

Increasing the cleansing frequency from every other day (Study #1) to 3 days on, 1 day off (Study #2) yielded 57% better results in ATEC changes.

Study #1 – average ATEC reduction was 35%
Study #2 – average ATEC reduction was 55%

All age groups responded very well:

Teenagers: Average ATEC reduction was 64%
Ages 10–12: Average ATEC reduction was 57%
Ages 4–9: Average ATEC reduction was 45%

Gender comparison:

Males: Average ATEC reduction was 58%
Females: Average ATEC reduction was 50%

All 27 participants experienced reductions in ATEC.

Cannabis

Using cannabis as an autism treatment is controversial. I haven't tried it for David, so I don't have firsthand experience with this intervention. Seizure disorders are disproportionately high among people with autism. When prescription drugs can't manage a seizure disorder, many parents turn to cannabis as an alternative to anti-seizure medications. I've met countless parents who have successfully reduced their children's seizures using cannabis. A few parents I met moved here to Colorado because their children were seizing up to 80 times per day. The seizures either subsided or were decreased to one or two small seizures per week shortly after cannabis was introduced.

If you are considering this as a treatment option, there is good information available from the group Mothers Advocating Medical Marijuana for Autism (MAMMA).[16] Another great source of information on CBD (short for cannabidiol) is from the late Dr. John Hicks. He researched CBD and its health benefits extensively and wrote a book called *The Medicinal Power of Cannabis.* His presentation at AutismOne (annual autism conference) may be helpful to parents as well. The link is in the endnotes.[17]

Marijuana is legal in Colorado. It's legal recreationally and for medicinal purposes. The use of medical marijuana is common here, and although we can't produce studies (The FDA will not allow clinical studies as it is still a federally controlled substance), the word on the street (by "street" I mean autism conferences I go to) is CBD, not necessarily THC, is most effective in our kids. CBD should not have the psychoactive properties of THC and, theoretically, will not give your child the sensation of being high. It is used strictly for repairing damage to the endocannabinoid system. It is greatly improving the lives of children with seizure disorders and parents of children with autism are reporting an increase in speech and socialization in their children. As with everything else, however, there is a great deal of individual variation, and what works for one child will not necessarily work for another. It can take a bit of time to find the best options for your child.

Essential oils

I am still learning about essential oils, but many parents of kids with autism have had great success. Again, David is doing so well that I don't necessarily need to add interventions to our routine, but my other two kids? Well, that's a different story. My youngest son Brooks is a firecracker. He's very headstrong and feisty as can be. Although I love and relate to his Viking nature, I have had to come up with creative ways to manage his intense behaviors.

I have used Peace and Calming (from Young Living) oil for him, and it really did help to settle him down. I also diffuse lavender essential oil when he gets worked up, and it almost immediately calms him down. I have tried frankincense in the diffuser a few times when he gets anxious and it seemed to help a bit, too.

Essential oils seem to have many benefits. I dug up an article from 2012, written by a mother whose son had pervasive developmental disorder (PDD), oppositional defiance disorder (ODD), and ADHD. She had immediate success with Valor (also Young Living) essential oil and decided she would use essential oils and supplements to reverse all diagnoses in her son.

She used several essential oils including Valor, lavender, Release, Brain Power, Citrus Fresh, and frankincense. The article explains how she used the oils and where she applied them on her son. After a few months her son recovered from his diagnoses and peace was restored in her home.[18]

Comorbid or co-occurring conditions

Comorbid conditions, sounds scary right? That's why many people have begun using the term "co-occurring" instead. Either way it means other medical conditions your child with autism may have. For example, David's comorbid conditions have included asthma, allergies, absence seizures (that went away after chelation), and chronic diarrhea. Previously, I mentioned underlying medical conditions; comorbid and co-occurring are just different words for this.

Common co-occurring conditions are Lyme and PANDAS or PANS. Lyme disease is common among our kids and is rather difficult to treat. Symptoms of Lyme are extensive but can include, muscle weakness or pain, confusion and memory loss, anxiety, psychosis, lightheadedness, blurred vision, and twitching of facial or other muscles. Lyme disease can look like many other illnesses and often goes undiagnosed. A brilliant autism mama I know, told me to test for Lyme using the DNA Connexions test.[19] She also said I can order an additional strep marker to test for co-infections. I haven't done the test yet because I just found out *how* to test for Lyme. I need to do it for David. I will order the test for David because I need to look at the results pertaining to viral infections, parasites, candida, and his ability to detox mercury. He is so close to full recovery, and I think this test can help me determine which steps I need to take next.

PANDAS is another condition that can occur in our kids. PANDAS is short for *p*ediatric *a*utoimmune *n*europsychiatric *d*isorders *a*ssociated with *s*treptococcal infections—say that five times fast. Let's just call it PANDAS or PANS, short for *p*ediatric *a*cute-onset *n*europsychiatric syndrome. These disorders can be tested for using the DNA Connexions tests, as they check for strep infections if you choose to add it to the testing. PANDAS Physicians Network also recommends testing the following if you feel your child may have PANS:

When evaluating a child for PANS:

1. Evaluate for Group A streptococcal infection.
2. Rule out acute rheumatic fever (echocardiography may be helpful)
3. Check for other infections.
4. Exclude non-infectious triggers.
5. Refer parents to a specialist.

The symptoms of PANS are:

1. Abrupt onset or abrupt recurrence of OCD or Restrictive Eating Disorder
2. Co-morbid neuropsychiatric symptoms (at least 2) with a similarly acute onset: anxiety, sensory amplification or motor abnormalities, behavioral regression, deterioration in school performance, mood disorder, urinary symptoms and/or sleep disturbances
3. Symptoms are not better explained by a known neurologic or medical disorder[20]

If I could do it all over again

If I could start over I would have approached David's recovery differently. I have spent about $800 per month on his diet, supplements and out-of-pocket professionals for about eleven years. It adds up to well over $100,000. not including insurance co-pays toward his therapy and doctor's visits.

If I could start over I would still do traditional methods of chelation because David's metals were so high. I would have done the diet and chelation and bought an IonCleanse to help his body detox. The IonCleanse is noninvasive; it helps with yeast overgrowth in the gut and helps to decrease the toxic body burden.

If I could start over I would not take the criticism of people who hadn't recovered a child to heart. Many doctors criticized and belittled me for putting him on the diet, but he is now their only patient to have (nearly) recovered. Some family members scoffed at me for putting him on the diet, but my son can tell me he loves me now. No one, not even me, can articulate what that means to me. I would have laughed more and worried less. My son is coming back to me; he is now a part of my world, and I wish I'd enjoyed his childhood more. Truth be told, this is why I'm writing this book. Your child deserves their childhood and deserves for the people taking care of him or her to be happy. I want you and your child to be happy and sometimes the only way to achieve that is through biomedical interventions. People will doubt you; they will scoff at you. Pay them no mind. Someday your child could be thriving and able to communicate with you, and it will all be worth it. Never give up.

THEN AND NOW, STORIES OF RECOVERY

Recovery is a sticking point in the autism community. I've heard of people with autism being frustrated by the word "recovery." But we don't seek recovery because we don't accept our kids the way they are or because we don't think they're perfect as they are. People with autism are the best, and in all honesty, I often prefer to be around people on the spectrum over typical people. I love them. On top of that, I basically worship the ground David walks on. He's the best kid I could hope for, and he has autism. Recovery isn't about changing your beautiful child, it's about addressing their underlying medical conditions and getting them well enough to care for themselves when you no longer can.

The reason that I am working to recover David is simple: When I'm gone, I am not sure who will take care of him.

Maybe other people have big families or in-laws who will take their children, but I really don't know who would be able to keep up with David's constant therapies and doctors' appointments, fight with the schools, address his tendency to wander off, and monitor his asthma, allergies, and diet. There are people in my life who love David; but loving him is not the same thing as caring for him.

We did a video for the Autism Society of Colorado some years ago. The videographer asked David, "What is autism?" To which David responded, "It's the greatest." Then the man asked, "What is it like to have autism?" and David said, "Really hard." The last question broke my heart; the videographer said, "What is the hardest part of having autism?" and David replied, "No friends."

No friends...that kills me. He is the coolest, nicest, most compassionate guy in the world. He's handsome and smart. He should have all the friends in the world. If my choosing biomedical interventions for him means that he can someday have friends and a better life, then it was all worth it. Every penny, every hour I spend preparing meals and wandering around the grocery store in search of new foods is worth it if it means my son will have a better quality of life.

If we're talking about full recovery from autism, my son is not an example of that. He's 90% better than he was when we started. That being said, most of us will take a 90% improvement and be glad. This section, however, isn't about 90% better; it's about complete and total recovery from autism.

Recovery is possible, and I think we're almost there. Keep in mind, David's autism was as severe as it gets, he didn't have ABA therapy when he was younger, and he wasn't diagnosed until he was almost five (doctors said his symptoms were too severe to be autism and felt he had a psychiatric disorder). Being diagnosed so late, he missed the window for early intervention services. Those things hindered his progress, but even today, as I write this chapter, I have complete and total confidence that he will be fine in a year or two.

Our biomedical journey has been twelve years long. Some parents get their kids recovered in two years or less. I know now after years of research that the severity of David's symptoms and behaviors before the interventions is exceedingly rare. Odds are your child is starting from a significantly better place than he did, and odds are you'll have an easier time at recovery than we did.

There are countless kids who've recovered, and I can't tell each family's story (although I'd like to), so I've selected a few to share with you. These kids didn't start out "high-functioning," and they weren't diagnosed with Asperger's. The children in the following examples had two things in common: classic autism and parents who refused to give in, also known as "warrior parents."

There are many stories of full recovery on the TACAnow. org website as well as at generationrescue.org. I've chosen only a few for the book, but all stories of recovery have the same result: The child is no longer on the autism spectrum. The choice to work toward recovery is yours and yours alone. Because I know your doctor will tell you that it is impossible for your child to lose the diagnosis of autism, I feel it is only right that someone tell you it is possible. It generally takes therapy combined with biomedical interventions to make that seemingly impossible dream of recovery a reality. Remember, David now says, "I love you." These are words I never thought I would hear from my son, and those words—that mean more to me than anything in the world—are possible because of biomedical interventions and ten years of therapy.

Quinn

Quinn was meeting his milestones and was on track in terms of his development. At 12 months, he received his MMR vaccine, and shortly after came the symptoms of autism. At 25 months, he was diagnosed with mild-to-moderate autism. He no longer responded to his name and had constant ear infections, eczema, diaper rash that never went away, loose stools, problems sleeping, dark shadows under his eyes, and often tried to elope.

Quinn's parents did research online and thought that a change in diet might be beneficial. They started by removing milk (casein): "Taking Quinn off of milk made a huge difference within only a few days—it was like he came out of a fog. He was more social and engaging than he'd ever been. He seemed happier."

Quinn's mom knew that there were solutions and that there was hope. Her research enabled her to find solutions:

> I clung to the anchor of hope that other parents had given us, and our journey into biomedical interventions began. We then changed his diet to be gluten-free/casein-free (GFCF), and he continued to improve. We found an experienced Defeat Autism Now! (DAN!) doctor to help us.

Quinn's parents made sure he had the right therapies in addition to vitamins and supplements he needed for optimal health. They kept up with the recommendations from the DAN! (now called MAPS) doctor and were meticulous in their approach to recovery. In the end, their hard work paid off. Quinn is now fully recovered and has lost the diagnosis of autism.

His story is similar to other children who have recovered. It takes dedication and perseverance, but it can happen!

> At the end of kindergarten during his triennial IEP, Quinn scored in the 93rd percentile for his age in speech. In first grade, on the Iowa Test of Basic Skills, Quinn's core total score was in the 79th percentile, and on the language subtest he scored in the 98th percentile. The test report read, "Language seems to be an area of relative strength for Quinn."

Quinn's story of recovery can be found on the TACA website or you can follow the link at the end of the book. There are many inspiring stories of recovery on this website. I would recommend looking at these stories to see if any of them resonate with you. The stories of recovery are all a little different and reading through them may help you to determine which course of action may work best for your family.[21]

Clay

In the book, *A Child's Journey out of Autism*, Leann Whiffen tells the story of her son Clay's descent into the world of autism and her and her husband's journey to pull him back out.

I highly recommend reading this book as it details life with autism and the miracle of recovery. Leann and her husband Sean were fully committed to getting their son as healthy as they could. Recovery was a long journey for Clay and his family, but in the end, determination got the better of autism. Clay is now recovered and is living the life he deserves to live, the life of a healthy child.

Clay's story is very similar to other families. Leann asked the doctor about recommended vaccines, to which he replied (while shaking and pointing his finger at her), "Mrs. Whiffen, Clay is much more likely to get smallpox than autism." (Note: We stopped vaccinating for smallpox in the 1970s, and it was declared eradicated from the *world* in 1980.) Leann, like most of us, was made to feel stupid and inferior when asking about vaccines. Reluctantly, she allowed Clay to get vaccinated.

In the months that followed, Clay would have bouts of smelly green diarrhea alternating with constipation. He would often bang his head or spin the wheels on his truck and had little eye contact and severe tantrums.

After going through their biomedical protocol, Leann and Sean can now say that their son is recovered:

> Clay is a typical third grade boy—not even his teacher knows of his past.... He is no longer on a gluten and casein free diet and takes just a daily multivitamin. He truly believes that there isn't anything wrong in the world. His pure, optimistic attitude serves as the framework for the family."[22]

These children are just a few examples of kids who've recovered from autism. As I read these stories, I can't help but think of the subtitle of the book *Autism: Effective Biomedical Treatments,* by Sidney Baker and Jon Pangborn: *"Have We Done Everything We Can for This Child?"* The truth is that David is not fully recovered, and I haven't done everything I can for him. I haven't tested him for Lyme or strep, and I need to take him in and run more viral panels. Until we can say we have done everything we can for our child, there is never a reason to abandon hope of recovery or vast improvement.

Daniel

Daniel's story changed everything for us. If for no other reason, it gave me the hope I needed to move forward. Daniel's story is similar to many of our children's stories. He had chronic green diarrhea, he stopped playing peekaboo, stopped walking, and stopped engaging with his family. Daniel banged his head on walls and writhed in pain on the ground. His symptoms were so similar to my own son's that I knew the answers I was looking for were in the article written by his mother.

Daniel's mother, who is now my real-life friend and hero, Mary Romaniec, wrote this article in hopes that other desperate parents would find answers in her child's story of regression and recovery. Her son's story was my son's story, and I knew if she could heal her son, I could heal mine. She emphasizes the importance of diet and her words have stayed with me:

> But in less than a week of eating no dairy prod-
> ucts Daniel stopped waking up screaming after
> his naps. Inspired, I stopped feeding him wheat
> as well, though only half-heartedly....Finally, we
> buckled down, committed 100 percent to Daniel's
> new diet, and saw a huge change in his behavior.
> But after three weeks on the diet, we blew it, vac-
> illating a little here and a little there. After a few
> weeks of this, Daniel was in full regression.[23]

I learned from Mary's story that there are no vacations from the diet and cross-contamination was not an option either. I stuck to the diet and watched my son flourish. Daniel's story has been an inspiration to me, and even today he is doing remarkably well. Daniel is in his first year of college and is doing exceptionally well in math. He has a bright future ahead of him, all thanks to his parent's diligence and refusal to give up hope.

EMBRACING A CHANGING LIFESTYLE

If you decide to go through with biomedical interventions, your life will change dramatically. Yes, in most cases your child will start to improve, and life will get easier after a month or two, but that's not the change I'm talking about. I'm talking about the changes that will occur as a result of putting your child on the diet.

If you choose to go through with the diet, be prepared. Every person you meet will now be a dietician, giving you lots of unsolicited advice. You'll hear things like: "He won't get enough calcium if you take him off milk. What about his bones?" "He's a kid. It's mean to not let him eat cake and ice cream." "What are you going to do about birthday parties?"

You can tell the dietician to cool it—there are solutions. Regarding calcium, coconut milk actually has more calcium than cow's milk. There are a variety of milk products you can choose from, all containing adequate amounts of calcium. In addition, orange and other juices are often fortified with calcium. It's as simple as reading labels and calculating the amount of calcium per serving.

As far as "being mean" (which I've heard a hundred times with David), it's "meaner" to keep feeding a kid something that is making them sick. Most of the "bad" behavior associated with autism can be attributed to the fact that kids are in pain and cannot communicate their physiological symptoms to their parents. It's not mean to give your child gluten-free brownies and cake instead. It may take a while to adjust to the new flavors, but they get used to it. Our kids can still have "ice cream," but it is rice or coconut milk-based instead. They can still eat pizza, bread, and donuts, but it is all gluten and casein-free. Again, TACAnow.org can be your saving grace for recipes. They have really great ideas, all from moms and dads who have walked in your shoes.

When people ask me "What is he going to eat at a birthday party?", my answer is "I make cake and bring it with us." It's as simple as that. There are alternatives to the food your child is used to eating, and yes, they are likely to resist the diet at first, but like the rest of us, you and your child will get through the changes just fine.

Because the diet is a huge commitment, you'll want to give some thought as to how you'll handle the holidays. For most of us, holidays are a time to meet with family and eat a variety of different foods. My friend, for example, has an amazing family, and every holiday they *all* eat GF/CF foods. That is the ideal situation, to have the entire family on board, but because it's rare to have an entire family agree to go GF/CF, you'll need to strategize.

TACAnow.org has great (printable) information on the diet. It may be helpful to print some information out and get it to your family members before the holiday season starts. It helps to have a conversation about the diet beforehand because you'll want to avoid people accidentally feeding your child something that is not on the diet.[24]

It also helps to talk to your family and friends about the diet and about autism in general because the majority of people are good willed. Most people want to help and be supportive of you and your child, but they don't know how. Information is empowering. Give them the opportunity to be empowered and to feel like they are able to contribute to your child's success in some small way. The goal is to set the holidays up for success.

I find it helpful to keep digestive enzymes in my purse for accidental dietary infractions, especially on the holidays. I will give David enzymes immediately if he eats foods that he shouldn't have, and although he still regresses a little bit, the enzymes stop him from having regressing and losing skills. He is still highly sensitive to foods. Separate from his gluten and casein intolerances, his food allergies are a serious health issue and infractions cannot be remedied with enzymes. The enzymes are not a cure-all, but they can help keep your child from having a full-blown regression if they eat the dreaded gluten or casein.

Another thing you'll want to consider in your changing lifestyle is how you'll address the diet issue with your family. Speaking from experience, it can be difficult until they see the progress your child makes on the diet—and the regressions they experience if they come off of it. It was particularly hard in my family because when I put David on the diet, we were living with my parents, and I had little control over the food that was in the house.

David would sneak food from the cupboards, and I had no way to control his access to food. After several attempts I was finally able to get David GF/CF for a solid 30 days, and the results were staggering. He was making better eye contact, his tantrums were almost gone, and he was starting to speak. Once my mom saw the progress he was making, she was on board. And thank God she was. My mom was my greatest asset through the first few months of the diet.

My mom read countless articles and books on diet and came up with clever ways to make David's food taste delicious. It wasn't until she saw his remarkable improvement that she recognized the value of the diet. My mom was a hard sell on the diet in the beginning. Being Italian, she thought it was ludicrous to remove pasta and bread from his diet!

The best thing you can do in this regard is to educate your family. You can print out information from the web or photocopy pages out of a book you found helpful. There are ways to be proactive and for this to be a positive experience for everyone involved.

If, however, you have a family member who lets your child sneak food, you may have to be the bad guy and not let your child go with that person for a considerable amount of time. I've done it, and it wasn't fun, but neither was cleaning up diarrhea and watching my son slip back into the world of autism. I have the attitude that, yes, I am the bad guy sometimes, but it is for my son's benefit. And if someone doesn't like it, I hope they don't let the door hit them on the way out.

Another consideration with the diet is school. If you see a MAPS doctor or you have a doctor who sees the value in the diet, you can ask them for a letter stating that the child is not allowed to have gluten or casein. The letter goes in your child's school file, and if they have a medical or health plan included in their IEP, the letter will be included in their file. I have added David's diet to his IEP, and I actually have stipulated that he only eat what I send. I provide a list of allowable foods for school parties and events in case I miss something.

THINGS YOU SHOULD KNOW BEFORE YOU VACCINATE

Vaccines are a part of American culture; it's just something we do. When I put David's medical file in chronological order and realized vaccines triggered his autism, I was devastated—emotionally, spiritually, and mentally devastated. I took David's medical file to his pediatrician and said, "I figured out what caused David's autism. I'm not going to say a word. I want you to read through his file and see if you notice what I noticed."

After a few minutes the pediatrician turned white as a ghost and began shaking. He stumbled over to his file drawer, started fumbling around and said, "You signed the piece of paper saying you can't sue me right?" I said, "Yes, I signed it. I know I can't sue you, and I can't sue the manufacturer." At the end of the day, if your child is injured by a vaccine, please know you can't sue the doctor who administered the vaccine(s) or the pharmaceutical companies that made them. It is a liability-free industry. My son's pediatrician was not at all concerned about David's quality of life, his future, his loss of language, or his chronic diarrhea; he was only concerned for himself. Not only did the pediatrician show no remorse for what happened to David, his immediate concern was money. Wow! I thought you were in my corner, dude. Guess not.

Vaccines are something we just do. Most of us don't think about them. We don't read up on ingredients; we show up, get our kids vaccinated, and leave after feeding our baby high-fructose corn syrup suckers or lollipops as a reward from the pediatrician. When David stopped speaking after his MMR and developed explosive, chronic diarrhea, I still didn't question vaccines. I was *sure* vaccines had been thoroughly studied for safety. I was *sure*—without researching vaccines—that our government had stringent regulations and that the CDC was an independent agency with no ties to pharmaceutical companies. I was wrong on all counts.

Before you rush to judgment and throw this book across the room, please know that most of us were once pro-vaccine and *knew* vaccines were safe and effective. If you can read through the list below and still feel comfortable vaccinating, by all means do so. Vaccines, like any other medical procedure, come with risks, and unlike the average medical procedure, vaccines do not require prior informed consent. Parents deserve and should have the right to know the risks associated with vaccines *before* entering into a potentially life-changing medical procedure. So here it is, things you should know before you vaccinate.

Before we get deeply into to this heated subject, I think it's important to hear from one of my heroes and the father of biomedical interventions, the late Dr. Bernard Rimland:

STATEMENT BY BERNARD RIMLAND, PH.D.
Director, Autism Research Institute
Editor, Autism Research Review International
Founder, Autism Society of America
THE AUTISM EPIDEMIC IS REAL, AND EXCESSIVE VACCINATIONS ARE THE CAUSE

The vaccine manufacturers, the Center for Disease Control, the FDA, and the various medical associations have failed miserably in their duty to protect our children. Rather than acknowledge their role in creating the immense, catastrophic rise in autism, these organizations have resorted to denial and obfuscation. They stand to lose their credibility, and billions of dollars in liability suits will soon reach the courts.

As a full-time professional research scientist for 50 years, and as a researcher in the field of autism for 45 years, I have been shocked and chagrined by the medical establishment's ongoing efforts to trivialize the solid and compelling evidence that faulty vaccination policies are the root cause of the epidemic. There are many consistent lines of evidence implicating vaccines, and no even marginally plausible alternative hypotheses.

As the number of childhood vaccines has increased 700%, from 3 in the '70s to 22 in 2000, the prevalence of autism has also showed a parallel increase of 700%.

Late onset autism, (starting in the 2nd year), was almost unheard of in the '50s, '60s, and '70s; today such cases outnumber early onset cases 5 to 1, the increase paralleling the increase in required vaccines.

Thousands of parents report—and demonstrate with home videos—that their children were normal and responsive until suffering an adverse vaccine reaction. (The Autism Research Institute has been tracking such autism-related vaccination reactions since 1967.)

Mercury, one of the most toxic substances known, is used as a preservative in many vaccines. Some infants have had 125 times the maximum allowable limit of mercury injected directly into their bloodstreams, in one day, in vaccines. (People vary enormously in their sensitivity to mercury, because certain genes predispose to mercury sensitivity. The highly-touted New England Journal of Medicine Danish study failed to mention the very convenient fact that none of the Danish children had prior exposure to mercury, since Denmark, unlike the U.S., had banned mercury from childhood vaccines in 1992, the year before the birth year of the children in the study.

There are numerous scientific studies showing large differences in clinical laboratory measures of blood, urine and biopsies which compare autistic children with normal controls. Such findings, pointing directly to vaccines as the cause of the group differences, are conveniently overlooked by those attempting to conceal the strong connection between the autism epidemic and excessive use of unsafe vaccines.

The truth must—and will—emerge. It is long over-due.[25]

1. There has never been a large-scale study comparing the health outcomes of vaccinated vs. completely unvaccinated children. My generation had 20 vaccines by age 18; kids now get 72 vaccines by age 18. There has never been a study that looks at the safety of the full vaccine schedule or looks at health outcomes of children who receive 72 vaccines by age 18.

2. There have been no studies on synergistic toxicity. Synergistic toxicity is the toxic burden of combining two or more ingredients together. For example, some vaccines contain mercury-based Thimerosal, though it has been "removed" from many childhood vaccines, it remains in most flu vaccines given to pregnant women and children over six months of age. Some vaccines contain aluminum, Professor Boyd Haley explains:

> We have demonstrated the toxicity of thimerosal by using it to kill neurons in culture. At 50 nanomolar thimerosal the neuron killing capacity/rate is about doubled with the addition of levels of aluminium found in vaccines. The aluminium alone at this level is not demonstrated to be toxic, so it is enhancing the toxicity of the thimerosal. It likely does this by increasing the rate that thimerosal breaks down releasing ethylmercury which is the toxic material.[26]

3. Members of the Advisory Committee on Immunization Practices (ACIP), which is responsible for determining which vaccines are "recommended" (states often use these "recommendations" to determine which vaccines to "require" for children to attend school), often work for pharmaceutical companies (who manufacture vaccines) and add vaccines to the schedule while on the payroll for both the government *and* pharmaceutical companies. Basically, in some instances pharmaceutical company employees add vaccines to the schedule, which frequently become "mandatory." What could go wrong?[27]

4. CDC employees often leave their positions at the CDC to work for pharmaceutical companies (vaccine manufacturers). For example, Julie Gerberding was the Director of the CDC from 2002-2009. Before leaving her position at the CDC, she produced a report on prevention of HPV that was probably instrumental in getting the FDA to fast-track the Gardasil HPV vaccine made by Merck, meaning that the vaccine went through a shortened approval process. Gerberding left the CDC to head up Merck's vaccine division.

Additionally, HPV vaccine studies did not use a true placebo. They used a solution containing an aluminum adjuvant instead of an inactive substance like saline. As a result, the studies showed little difference in adverse reactions between the HPV vaccine and the "placebo." HPV vaccines have been a cause for concern in the medical community. Dr. Sin Hang Lee has filed allegations of scientific misconduct with the World Health Organization (WHO) pertaining to this vaccine.

Julie Gerberding also presided over the CDC when it conducted studies exonerating the MMR vaccine (another Merck product) in the development of autism. As an executive at Merck, Gerberding has profited enormously from work she oversaw while at the CDC.[28]

5. Acetaminophen could actually be a driving force in the autism epidemic. Acetaminophen hinders the production of glutathione, and glutathione is needed to detox. In the U.S., we commonly give our children acetaminophen before or after vaccines which makes it extremely difficult for some patients to excrete toxic vaccine ingredients like mercury, aluminum, formaldehyde, ammonium sulfate, ethanol, etc. If the medical community were to acknowledge the deleterious effects of administering acetaminophen at the time of vaccination, they may make this product available by prescription only and we'd likely see a dramatic decrease in autism cases.[29]

6. Not all doctors think all vaccines are safe for all children. It is not uncommon for a person to get a second opinion when they are considering a medical procedure such as surgery. Vaccines are just another medical procedure, and there are many doctors who have concerns about long-term health outcomes of vaccinated children. It's worth getting a second opinion. There are many doctors speaking out about vaccine safety. I'll list a few so you can access another opinion: Dr. Nancy Banks, Dr. Suzanne Humphries, Dr. Toni Bark, Dr. Paul Thomas, Dr. Robert Sears (author of The Vaccine Book), Dr. Lawrence Palevsky, and others have done extensive research on vaccine safety and efficacy.[30] Many people are unaware that most doctors receive very little education on vaccine safety, synergistic toxicity and recognizing adverse reactions during medical school.

7. In 2014 Senior CDC Scientist, William Thompson, Ph.D., made the following statement:

> *I regret that my coauthors and I omitted statistically significant information in our 2004 article published in the journal Pediatrics. The omitted data suggested that African American males who received the MMR vaccine before age 36 months were at increased risk for autism.*[31]

Since 2004 an incalculable number of children have been diagnosed with autism. Unfortunately, Dr. Thompson has yet to be granted a Congressional hearing to investigate these allegations.

8. A few brave journalists are reporting on the connection between vaccines and autism. Sharyl Attkisson and Ben Swann have done great stories on the topic.[32]

9. Mercury-based Thimerosal was removed from pediatric vaccines (except trace amounts which do not have to be listed on the insert). Then the CDC recommended flu vaccines for pregnant women, and many flu vaccines still contain Thimerosal. The CDC also recommended the TDaP (tetanus, diphtheria, and pertussis) vaccine for pregnant women. TDaP contains aluminum, which is a known neurotoxin. There has never been a break in mercury and aluminum exposure in the pediatric population since the removal of mercury-based Thimerosal from pediatric vaccines.

10. The CDC itself has published reports showing that DTaP vaccination does not effectively prevent pertussis (whooping cough) infection. In the 2014 CDC Surveillance Report, the agency looked at efficacy rates of the DTaP vaccine; 41% (1,810) of the children who had contracted pertussis between the ages of one and four years had had all three recommended doses of the DTaP vaccine. This vaccine is given to children in the assumption that it will prevent pertussis infection, but, ummm...according to the CDC, even three doses of the vaccine does not always provide protection. When looking at the link provided, it appears that a child who receives this vaccine is just as likely to contract pertussis than those children who received zero doses.[33]

11. Vaccines have never been tested on pregnant women. Technically, the CDC and FDA don't know what these vaccines can do to a fetus. Mothers are the only source of data we have. If they have a miscarriage or their child has a birth defect, they are supposed to report it to the vaccine manufacturer. Doctors don't often tell pregnant mothers this, and these events often go unreported. In a recent article about VAXXED, a 2016 documentary about the CDC's efforts to discredit a study linking autism to the MMR vaccine, Dr. Katherine Hale stated, "I Saw VAXXED and I Was Shattered," Dr. Kathryn Hale, is an OB/GYN who also has a master's in Public Health, stated, "As physicians, we place our trust in organizations such as the CDC to give us the information we need to keep our patients safe. It changes you when you find that those you thought you could trust could not be trusted." She goes on to say, "After watching VAXXED, one thing is clear, there is a definite link between the MMR vaccine and autism. Children are being damaged and something needs to be done."[34] I am quoting this OB/GYN to drive home the fact that the doctors administering vaccines to pregnant women are starting to question the safety of these vaccines. If the CDC cannot be trusted to present fact-based data to doctors, we need to take a critical look at this agency and make immediate changes.

12. The amounts of aluminum and Thimerosal in vaccines exceed FDA safety guidelines. For example, the maximum amount of aluminum an 8-pound healthy baby can tolerate is 18.16 micrograms (mcg). The hepatitis B vaccine (given at birth) contains 225 mcg of aluminum. The FDA guideline for Thimerosal exposure is limited to 2 parts per billion (ppb) in drinking water; 200 ppb mercury in liquid waste is considered a toxic hazard; many flu vaccines contain 50,000 ppb.[35]

13. Injection and ingestion are two very different processes in the body. If a person ingests (eats) something toxic, the body has multiple avenues to rid itself of the toxin. If the toxin is injected, all the normal barriers are bypassed. My friend Shawn Siegel explains it best:

Reality: ingestion and injection are two completely different worlds. In fact, anything placed within the cavity of the human GI tract, technically speaking, is outside the body, a river that runs through it, while the capillary beds of the muscles, into which vaccines are deposited, and from which they're absorbed into the bloodstream, are deep inside. Much of what's ingested never reaches the bloodstream, and virtually all of what does has been significantly changed by the metabolic processes that take place in the cavity and walls of the GI tract and in the liver, before it enters the bloodstream.[36]

14. Doctors get very little education on vaccine safety in medical school. In fact, I've asked several pediatricians, who insisted David be caught up on his vaccines, "Who tells you vaccines are safe? Where do you get that information?" And they always answer the same way, "The CDC and the American Academy of Pediatrics (AAP)." My response is, "Well, a senior Scientist from the CDC says he knows vaccines are linked to autism, that the CDC pertussis surveillance report states even if my kids receive all the pertussis doses, they can still get pertussis, and that the AAP is partially funded by pharmaceutical companies. Can you give me a study to read? Which study are you basing your information on?" Not one pediatrician has been able to give me a study. One physician's assistant told me David needed to be caught up on his vaccines, and when I told her I wouldn't unless I could see the vaccinated vs. unvaccinated study, she said, "They did that study. How could they know vaccines were safe if they didn't?" My response was, "Ummm...yeah, that's what I'm saying. They have never done that study, and without having a third, independent party conduct that study, there is no evidence that vaccinated kids are healthier."

As I understand it, doctors are taught how to administer vaccines; they are told they are safe, and that's about it. If I understand this correctly, there is virtually nothing in the Symptoms and Diagnosis, Pathology, Biochemistry, Pathophysiology, Human Anatomy, Bates' Physical Exam,

EKG and Medical Interviews medical textbooks on vaccines. There is one paragraph in the Clinical Epidemiology medical textbook and one four-page chapter in the Microbiology textbook. Of about 6,700 pages doctors read in medical school, there are four pages on vaccines. Given the fact that vaccines are given by most doctors, it seems they should learn more about recognizing adverse reactions, synergistic toxicity, vaccine manufacturing and the possible negative effects of vaccinating while a child is sick. Doctors tell us to vaccinate and we assume they are the authority on vaccines. In my experience they actually know very little about vaccine safety and efficacy. That makes sense though. I've been researching vaccines for ten years now, and they have only read about four pages on the issue. It's what they don't know that is problematic.[37]

15. In a congressional hearing on the federal response to autism, the CDC representative, Dr. Coleen Boyle, was forced to admit they have never done a vaccinated vs. unvaccinated study. Oops. The link is in the endnotes if you care to watch it.[38]

16. One in 36 boys now has autism. Doctors and health agencies have no explanation as to why; they repeatedly say it's *not* vaccines. The increase in autism coincides with the increase in vaccines given to children.[39]

17. You can't sue a vaccine manufacturer if your child is injured or killed by a vaccine. If your child is injured by a vaccine, you will file with the Vaccine Injury Compensation Program (VICP), also known as "Vaccine Court," which is funded by taxpayers (a tax on each childhood vaccine sold goes to the compensation program). Vaccine manufactures can't be held liable in a court of law thanks to a 1986 federal law. When you take your child in to be vaccinated, you are probably not told you cannot sue a vaccine manufacturer (pharmaceutical company) if your child is injured. We, as U.S. citizens are at the mercy of pharmaceutical companies. We are banking on the idea they care more about us than profits. Considering the fact that Risperdal and Vioxx, among many other drugs, were put on the market, approved by the FDA, and *then* discovered to cause irreparable harm to people, that isn't very reassuring. Pharmaceutical companies have found a way to make enormous profits with no liability.

18. There is a database that tracks vaccine injury; if your child is injured by a vaccine, your doctor is supposed to report it to the Vaccine Adverse Event Reporting System (VAERS). Parents are not generally told this, and doctors rarely report vaccine injury. In my case, I know vaccines triggered my son's autism, and I have never reported it. It is estimated that only about 10% of vaccine injuries are ever reported to VAERS, which means that 90% of vaccine injuries go unreported.

19. As Americans, we credit vaccines for saving us from death from communicable diseases. However, if you look at these charts linked in the endnotes, you can see that death rates from these diseases sharply declined before their vaccines were introduced. Some diseases had virtually disappeared without the help of vaccines thanks to better plumbing and sanitation practices in the U.S.[40]

20. Polio, oh polio, the mother of vaccine debates. I'm not going to tackle this one. I'll let my brilliant friend, Shawn Seigel, take this one too. In the Notes section of his Facebook page he says the following:

> The year following the introduction of the polio vaccine, the CDC changed the diagnostic parameters of the disease, so drastically, that it automatically

eliminated two thirds of the cases of paralytic polio that would then be diagnosed.[41]

Not only were the diagnostic criteria for polio changed, but the polio vaccines themselves caused multiple deaths as well. The oral polio vaccine (OPV) and the inactivated polio vaccine (IPV) are available to the public, but we are not warned of the potential risks of these vaccines. Shawn goes on to say:

> *Meanwhile, between the OPV and the IPV, there have been over a thousand deaths reported to VAERS. While some of those reported deaths will likely prove unrelated to the vaccines, some of them will certainly prove directly, causally related—I assume most will, but that is beside this particular point, which is, numbers aside, the polio vaccine can kill.*[42]

What was once considered to be polio is now a host of illnesses, including meningitis.

> *Then there is the additional statistical issue of the re-diagnosis of cases of non-paralytic cases of polio as aseptic meningitis—and, I assume, other diseases that display similarly to non-paralytic polio.*[43]

When people tell me David needs to be vaccinated because polio might resurface, I tell them (1) he was vaccinated for polio, and (2) the definition of polio has changed so many times, it's unlikely the vaccine had the impact we were told it did.

> *In total, the diagnostic changes could easily account for as much as a 90% decline in the reported incidence of polio. In the subsequent years, however,*

as the CDC has pointed to the eradication of polio as one of the largest feathers in the cap of vaccination....[44]

The point of all this is that what we are told about vaccines and the truth are two very different things. It appears that vaccines may not have been responsible for "eradicating" polio, while the CDC changing the diagnostic criteria may have been. But wait, it gets worse:

In 1960 Bernice Eddy, a government researcher, discovered that when she injected hamsters with the kidney mixture on which the [polio] vaccine was cultured, they developed tumors.[45]

Did the CDC recall and destroy the vaccine? Nope:

Alarm spread through the scientific community as researchers realized that nearly every dose of the vaccine had been contaminated. In 1961 federal health officials ordered vaccine manufacturers to screen for the virus and eliminate it from the vaccine. Worried about creating a panic, they kept the discovery of SV40 under wraps and never recalled existing stocks. For two more years millions of additional people were needlessly exposed—bringing the total to 98 million Americans from 1955 to 1963.[46]

In a nutshell, the CDC wanted the entire population vaccinated for polio. When they learned that the vaccine was contaminated with SV40, they didn't recall it.

21. Measles. I'll take this one. When I gave testimony at a Bill hearing in Colorado last year because Health and Human Services wanted to take over our vaccine exemptions, a representative for my state told me, "Thousands of children

died from measles last year." Herein lies the problem: the people passing laws pertaining to vaccines are given misrepresented information, including third-world death statistics on disease. Pharmaceutical companies have spent over three billion dollars lobbying Congress. They are inundating our representatives with misleading information. They tell our reps the measles, mumps, rubella (MMR) vaccine is well studied and claim science has disproven the link between vaccines and autism. They fail to mention that many of the studies are either funded by a pharmaceutical company or have been shown to have altered critical data. Pharmaceutical company lobbyists tell your representatives that the MMR vaccine does not cause autism, but forget to tell them that, at a minimum, 83 cases of vaccine-induced autism have been recognized by the federal government, and the true total is likely to be well over 500.[47] When pharmaceutical company lobbyists sit down with your state representatives, they fail to tell them one constitutionally significant piece of information about the MMR vaccine: The MMR vaccine is cultured with WI-38. I was horrified to learn that WI-38 are aborted fetal cells from 1962. As I understand it, no cell line should be used longer than 30 years. Additionally, the child's (aborted child) mother was a psychiatric patient. This was all very shocking to learn, and although I hate to relay the gory details, I think you should know what I wish someone had told me years ago.

Using WI-38 is problematic for two reasons. One, I feel it violated my and my son's constitutional rights to practice our religion. I would not and cannot give any of my children vaccines containing aborted fetal cells because of my beliefs. It's not that I judge people who have had an abortion, because I don't. But for me, it's not on the table. As a Daughter of the American Revolution, my grandfathers and uncles fought for my Constitutional right to practice my religion. The First Amendment reads:

> *Congress shall make no law respecting an estab-*
> *lishment of religion or prohibiting the free exer-*
> *cise thereof; or abridging the freedom of speech,*
> *or of the press, or the right of the people peace-*
> *ably to assemble, and to petition the government*
> *for redress of grievances.*

David and I were denied informed consent (something that does not apply to vaccines), which in turn denied us our First Amendment right to practice our religion. I was not given the vaccine package insert for the MMR and did not have the opportunity to read the ingredients beforehand. Because David was injured by vaccines, he lost language. One could even make an argument that because of laws requiring vaccines he lost his right to free speech. Not only was I denied informed consent, vaccines also denied him his constitutional rights.

The second major concern about the use of WI-38 to make the MMR is the introduction of foreign DNA to our bodies. When we introduce foreign DNA it usually enters the body in the form of viruses, our bodies reject it and fight it. If that DNA is human, it can cause the body to turn on itself.

At the end of the Bill hearing, I stated that I was denied the freedom to practice my religion, and as a Christian I was upset to learn the MMR and many other vaccines contained these fetal cells. A few of the legislators scoffed at me when I said that. Here I am, the mother of a chronically ill, disabled child, and my own representatives scoffed at me for asserting my Constitutional rights (the same reps who cited third-world statistics). I am a registered Democrat, and their mocking me was enough to change my tune. I don't know how I'll vote in the years ahead, but I certainly won't vote for candidates who mock children with disabilities and their mothers.[48]

Unfortunately, our representatives have been given very little fact-based information on vaccine safety, efficacy, and ingredients. They are told they are safe, well studied, and there is no link between vaccines and autism. Their sources of information are typically the news (which relies on pharmaceutical company dollars), doctors (who rely on the CDC for public health recommendations), the American Academy of Pediatrics (who also benefit from pharmaceutical company dollars), and pharmaceutical company lobbyists.

In order to pass sound laws pertaining to public health and safety, our representatives must first have unbiased studies and data on vaccines. At present our representatives are where I was eleven years ago. They believe, like most of us parents did, that the CDC is an independent public health agency. Robert F Kennedy, Jr., described it best when he said:

> Public health may not be the sole driver of CDC decisions to mandate new vaccines. Four scathing federal studies, including two by Congress, one by the US Senate, and one by the HHS Inspector General, paint CDC as a cesspool of corruption, mismanagement, and dysfunction with alarming conflicts of interest suborning its research, regulatory, and policymaking functions. CDC rules allow vaccine industry profiteers like Dr. Offit to serve on advisory boards that add new vaccines to the schedule.[49]

22. Mississippi's infant mortality rates compare to those of third-world countries. On top of that, Mississippi has exceptionally high vaccination rates and exceedingly high rates of diabetes. The state has some of the highest premature and cancer-related deaths in the country. They also are high in deaths from cardiovascular disease. An article from the Washington Postclaims parents who worry about vaccine safety need not be concerned because, "Medical authorities have discredited these safety concerns."[50] They

don't cite any source to indicate which studies were used to "discredit" safety concerns. Did they use the study in which "Tom Verstraeten of the CDC modeled an association between neurologic developmental disorders and exposure to the mercury-based Thimerosal"? Is that what the Washington Post was referring to? I don't know because they didn't cite any sources. That study was published as a neutral study that didn't show anything either way. Yet earlier Verstraeten had written to his co-workers about his findings in an email titled "It just won't go away," referring to the strong, statistically significant correlation he was seeing between early high doses of Thimerosal and autism. And it's the same study that prompted a secret meeting at the Simpsonwood Conference Center in Norcross, GA, that was attended by pharmaceutical representatives where he said, "As you'll see some of the RRs [relative risks] increase over the categories and I haven't yet found an alternative explanation."[51] If publications are going to claim vaccines are safe, it sure would be nice if they cited their sources.

Some may argue that the poor health of Mississippi's residents may be attributed in part to diet and lifestyle choices. However, given the fact that their population is highly vaccinated, it begs the question, are vaccines contributing to the poor health of Mississippi's residents? The problem is always the same. Media outlets continuously use scare tactics, hoping we won't do any research of our own. The Disneyland measles outbreak is a perfect example. There was more false reporting on that than I can tackle right now, but one media outlet stated, "The point of the [MMR] vaccine is to prevent deaths from measles, mumps, and rubella like the recent episode of child deaths in California." But, there *were* no deaths from that measles outbreak. None at all. Yet, last year alone, 23 kids with autism died from wandering. There were more autism-related deaths last year than measles deaths in decades, but I guess the media isn't concerned about our babies.[52]

As I write this I have to remember how discouraged and angry I was when I figured out the autism/vaccine connection. Yes, I do think that vaccines triggered my son's autism, but how it happened is complex and took me years to fully understand. There are countless books on the subject, such as *Evidence of Harm, Callous Disregard, Vaccine Epidemic, Dissolving Illusions, Thimerosal: Let the Science Speak: The Evidence Supporting the Immediate Removal of Mercury—a Known Neurotoxin—from Vaccines,* and *Vaccine Whistleblower,* to name a few. There are many documentaries on the topic, including *The Greater Good, Vaxxed* (about the CDC whistleblower), *Silent Epidemic, Trace Amounts, The Truth about Vaccines, Vaccines Revealed,* and *Bought.*

Are vaccines the *only* cause of autism? Probably not. Acetaminophen at the time of vaccination must be a driving force in the autism epidemic. If your child, like mine, has the MTHFR genetic mutation, they can't detox properly and are at an increased risk for autism once vaccinated. Genetically modified foods (GMOs) are also a probable cause. Dr. Stephanie Seneff from MIT has done extensive research on the topic, and she believes GMOs are a causal factor in the epidemic. The chart linked in the endnotes shows an increase in cases of autism beginning at the time GMOs were introduced into our food supply.[53]

The causes of autism are complicated and include both genetic and environmental components, but the recent tremendous rise in incidence is clearly being driven by environmental exposures. It is, in many cases, a man-made epidemic. Another problem is that Monsanto (the chemical company that produces GMOs and glyphosate) has an enormous amount of money and they use it to buy influence. An ex-Monsanto vice president, Michael Taylor, headed the FDA. Monsanto is a contributor to the Clinton Foundation, and President Trump met with Monsanto executives even before his inauguration. In addition, his Attorney General, Jeff Sessions, appears likely to approve a Monsanto-Bayer merger, making it one of the world's biggest agriculture conglomerates. Getting Monsanto out of our government is the only way we can get the FDA to properly research the deleterious effects of GMOs and glyphosate[54] on the population.

The other issue is the amount of influence pharmaceutical companies and large corporations like Monsanto have on our government. People understand our government is corrupt in some ways: The banks got a bailout and we got the bill. Insurance companies are allowed to charge unnecessarily high prices for drugs. They "misplaced" trillions of dollars in 2001. The list goes on and on. People understand instinctively that there are issues with government corruption, but they want to believe that the one thing they wouldn't mess up is vaccines. I hate to be the bearer of bad news, but they messed that up too.

Vaccines are big business, and with no liability there is no incentive to be cautious about adding vaccines to the schedule. My generation had few cases of autism with twenty doses of vaccines recommended by age eighteen. American children today are the least healthy they have ever been, and now seventy-two doses of vaccines are recommended by age eighteen. One in thirty-six boys now has autism, and one in six American children now has a developmental disability. By one mainstream estimate, half of American children are suffering from chronic illnesses. There are over two hundred vaccines in the pipeline. If pharmaceutical companies have their way, the federal government will mandate vaccines, and we could be forced to take countless vaccines with the manufacturers having no financial liability if (when) we're injured. This is not rocket science; clearly, vaccines are a contributing factor to the autism epidemic.

At the end of the day, what matters most are our children. Regardless of what causes autism, our focus must always be their well-being. Recovery from autism is repairing the damage of the environmental triggers that bring about symptoms we know as autism.

I know this information will make you angry. People have called me every name in the book for saying vaccines caused my son's autism, even though in my case his pediatrician acknowledged it. It brings out the worst in people because it's so scary. It's scary to think that what we've been told our entire lives is a lie. It's scary to think we can't trust our doctors. I actually feel bad for pediatricians because they have been given false information by the CDC. It's scary to think of what will happen if we stop vaccinating. It's scary, and fear often presents itself as anger.

This chapter will give you a good place to start on the road to recovery. If my son, who was considered "worst-case-scenario for autism", can, almost, recover, so can yours. Biomedical interventions are specific to the child, and in time you will find the interventions that work for your precious baby. Doctors told me David would never speak, he would never be in general education classes, and that I would have to institutionalize him. They were wrong on all counts.

In the famous words of Wilma Rudolph, "My doctors told me I would never walk again. My mother told me I would. I believed my mother." Have faith in yourself, believe you can do this, and you will. There will be hard days: Your child may kick your arse during the yeast die-off phase. They will resist the diet. There will be naysayers. Don't mind any of it, just visualize your child getting better, and in time they will. Never give up!

NOTES FOR CHAPTER 4

5

AUTISM-RELATED THERAPIES AND INTERVENTIONS

BEATITUDES FOR FRIENDS OF DISABLED CHILDREN

Blessed are you who take the time to listen to difficult speech, for you help us to know that if we persevere we can be understood.

Blessed are you who walk with us in a public place, and ignore the stares of strangers, for in your companionship we find havens of relaxation.

Blessed are you who never bid us to "hurry up" and more blessed are you who do not snatch our tasks from our hands and do them for us, for often we need time rather than help.

Blessed are you who ask for our help, for our greatest need is to be needed.

Blessed are you who stand beside us as we enter new and untried ventures, for our failures will be outweighed by the times when we surprise ourselves and you.

Blessed are you who help us with the graciousness of Christ, for often we need the help we cannot ask for.

Blessed are you when by all things you assure us that thing that makes us individuals is not in our peculiar muscles, nor in our wounded nervous systems, nor in our difficulties in learning, but in the God-given self which no infirmity can confine.

Rejoice and be exceedingly glad and know that you give us reassurances that could never be spoken in words, for you deal with us as God deals with all of His Children.

—Adapted from Andre Masse, CSE[1]

THIS POEM COMPLETELY changed my perspective on my son. Maybe for the first time in his life, I really thought about his need to be needed. It also changed how I saw therapy. I realized I wasn't sitting through hours of therapy every week merely to help him function in society; I was doing so to help him feel empowered and capable. I saw that patience, not discipline, was the key to his success.

While chapter 3 should help you get started on insurance and getting the financial piece of therapy covered, in this chapter, I will try to guide you through various therapy options. Remember, this can be a long process, and there are therapies and interventions listed in this chapter you can do at home while you're waiting for your insurance company to approve coverage. You don't have to have it all figured out immediately. Implement what you can at home, and in time, you will find the right therapies and the right therapists. It is like a marathon: You don't have to sprint to reach the finish line, you just have to keep going.

I didn't go to school for this, I received no formal training in autism-related therapies. I recognized early on that I needed advice from professionals. I needed people with experience and a fresh perspective to help my son learn everything from the activities of daily living and how to articulate sentences to how to advocate for himself.

Therapy is more than teaching our kids to sit quietly, use scissors, and participate in group activities. Therapy is designed to teach our kids the skills they need to care for themselves and to feel like they are contributing to the world around them. Ever since I read Andre Masse's poem, I started asking David for help. It started with little things like "Hand that to Mommy, please" or "You are better with electronics than I am (which is absolutely true). Can you please set up the video games for your brothers?" And I'd make a big deal about him helping me. The praise he received for assisting me made his chest puff up and his eyes beam. Because he was nonverbal at the time, people assumed he did not understand them and was therefore incapable of helping with small tasks. As time has gone on, David has been taught to unload the dishwasher and even do his own laundry. Every time he is asked for help, his face lights up, and he practically skips to do his chores, elated at the prospect of helping me solve a problem. He loves the feeling of being needed and having the ability to help his mama. His ability to complete household chores would have been next to impossible if not for biomedical interventions and occupational and behavior therapies.

The therapies your child participates in can change the direction of their life. Some of our kids may never live on their own, but a therapy program that includes behavior and speech therapy can help them communicate needs, wants, and interests. The ability to communicate will help to decrease negative behaviors and enable them to have input into their own lives. Some of our kids can live independently but will require good occupational and behavior therapists to teach them money management, safety skills, bus routes, and appropriate social behaviors needed to maintain employment.

Therapy can be a pain in the butt for parents. For the last thirteen years, my life has revolved around David's therapy schedule. Since age two he has had between two and three therapy sessions per week (occupational and speech therapy), and in the summer as many as five to six days every week. My son went from worst-case-scenario for autism to high-functioning thanks to my persistence, David's desire to get well, biomedical interventions—and therapy. There is no easy road. If your child is going to improve, it is going to take time, diligence, sacrifice, and a well thought-out, structured schedule that includes therapy.

I love David the way he is and watching him improve and getting to know my son has been like witnessing a miracle. He is so kind and sweet; he is generous, funny, and so smart. His experiences have shaped him into the exceptional human being he is today and have somehow made me a better, more compassionate person. His therapists, while teaching him essential life skills, have helped bring out the best in him.

Therapy, like most things, is what you make of it. I decided in the beginning that my job was to support the therapists in every way I could. I made sure that no matter what was going on in my personal life, I would be positive and encouraging to every therapist who walked through my front door. Although David went through a phase where he tore my house apart every day, I tried to make sure my house was clean, and his therapists had a clutter-free area to work in. I wanted to create a relaxing and peaceful environment for therapy.

Therapy can be a positive, fun, enjoyable learning experience for both the parents and child. Because there are so many therapies to choose from, I will summarize the many therapy options in the shortest way possible. This will give you a general idea of why the particular therapy or intervention is used as an autism treatment and whether it will benefit your little guy or girl. Let's get to it!

- Choose the best therapies and interventions for your child
- Know that you can change direction at any time. (As your child improves, the therapies can be adjusted or eliminated accordingly.)

CHOOSE THE BEST THERAPIES AND INTERVENTIONS FOR YOUR CHILD

There are a myriad of effective therapies you can choose from to help your child with ASD. However, early intervention is vital to your child's development. The sooner you can get started, the better. Not every child will have access to early intervention services, and in that case parents can apply core principles of the therapies listed below until insurance approves therapy.

David has had speech therapy, also known as *speech language pathology* (SLP) and *occupational therapy* (OT) since age two. He was recently discharged from OT as he has mastered all the skills they can teach him! A few years ago, we added behavioral therapy, which has been instrumental in increasing his safety awareness as well as helping to develop his social skills. I have done my own version of Son-Rise therapy at home and have worked side-by-side with his therapists to make sure I am reinforcing their suggestions at home.

Committing to a therapy schedule can be difficult. I've kept up with David's therapy schedule whether I was working full-time or staying home with him. It's not always easy, but well worth it in the end. When David's dad and I got divorced, I went back to work immediately. With my schedule I was able to keep him in speech after work one day a week, and OT came on the weekend. It was minimal, but it did help him establish a relationship with his therapists and gain beginning functional communication and skills pertaining to activities of daily living (ADLs).

No matter what is going on in our personal lives, therapy must always be a priority and everything else (but work and sometimes family) needs to become secondary to the therapy schedule. Honestly, autism can be very isolating and sometimes the only adults I talk to all week are his therapists. I actually look forward to seeing them and having an adult conversation, even if it's just for a few minutes.

Therapy is important and choosing the right **therapist** is key to your child's development. David has had about twelve speech therapists. I fired a few, most left on their own because he was so violent in the beginning, some left for personal reason and others simply didn't have the experience to help him gain skills. You may have to let some therapists go because they don't have the right experience or don't click with your child. Never feel bad about letting a therapist go. If they aren't a good fit, your child won't make gains and it will have been a waste of time and money. I have let many therapists go. I did so graciously and was considerate of their feelings, but I had to do what was best for my son. Sometimes doing what is best for David means I need to have uncomfortable conversations. This is not a popularity contest. Not everyone is going to like you or your decisions, and that is okay.

I would also like to stress the importance of trusting your gut instincts. If a new therapist gives you a bad feeling or your child seems anxious around that person, take that into consideration when deciding whether or not to keep them on board. Additionally, I have always been very hands-on with David. Therapy happens in my living room or in a room with the door open. I want to know what the therapist is working on and what strategies to implement at home. I don't think our kids being alone in a closed room with a stranger is a good idea; if the therapist wants to be in a closed room to reduce sensory stimulus, put a camera in the room. Nonverbal children are far more likely to be abused than their typical peers, and that needs to weigh into our decision-making process. I am not trying to make you apprehensive or anxious about therapy; I just think there need to be boundaries and parental involvement in all aspects of a therapy regimen. If a therapist makes you uncomfortable or it's not a good fit, let them go and find someone new. The next therapist may be the perfect person for your family. It is similar to love relationships in the sense that we can't make room for the perfect person if the wrong person is still hanging around.

Following are some of the therapies from which you can choose. Some are mainstream while others are more alternative (whatever that means), but you know your child best. You decide which therapies will benefit your child.

Wilbarger Brushing Technique

The Wilbarger Brushing Technique, "brushing" for short, is not exactly a therapy, but I am listing it first for a reason. Therapy can be very costly, and it may take time to get your pediatrician to sign a referral and/or your insurance company to cover the cost of therapy. The brushing technique is highly effective for kids with sensory issues and can be lifesaver for children who are struggling with sensory sensitivity. When David was about four, we started the brushing to help him de-escalate when he was on sensory overload (which was most of the time). He was resistant at first; he'd hit and kick me while I brushed him, but I persisted. After he was used to being brushed, he craved it, and eventually started bringing me his brush if he needed to calm down.

The brushing technique is used to decrease sensory sensitivity and seems to help our kids get centered. If you work with an OT, odds are they are familiar with this technique and can guide you with instruction, or you can ask your school's OT for training. The brushing technique must be done correctly, with joint compressions, if it is to be effective. I can't emphasize enough the importance of doing this correctly. I had David's former OT train the staff at his day care on how to brush him and do the joint compressions. One day I picked him up from day care, and he was off the charts. He was running around screaming, tearing up papers, hitting people, throwing toys, etc. I asked what they did differently that day, and the girl assigned to his room said, "I didn't do anything different. I brushed him for like twenty minutes, and now he's doing this."

Ummm...that is not how it works. Brushing him for twenty minutes overstimulated him and had the opposite of a calming effect. Brushing must be done with deep pressure, can only be done every 90-120 minutes (I stick to 120 to avoid overstimulation), and should be accompanied by joint compressions. I recommend seeking the advice of an OT because they are trained to accurately do joint compressions and can help you learn the proper methods of doing so.

Benefits of the Wilbarger Brushing Technique are:

BEHAVIORAL CHANGES

+ increased motivation
+ thinking before acting
+ increased open-mindedness
+ improved organization
+ improved sequencing (organized thinking, such as putting tasks in order)
+ improved focus
+ decreased sensitivity to smells
+ decreased sensitivity to touch
+ less irritability
+ better at beginning or completing projects
+ less behavioral rigidity
+ improved attention span
+ decreased hyperactivity
+ decreased impulsivity
+ improved transitions
+ increased participation in activities
+ improved interactions with peers

An OT can provide you with a brush. However, I know that hospitals, and sometimes produce departments, have the brushes available. The endnotes provide a link to purchase the brush online if you choose to do so.[2] Brushing is a great way to address sensory issues and is something you can do at home for a minimal price (the cost of a brush).

Speech therapy

Having a good speech therapist is worth more than gold. A good speech therapist can address the needs of your child wherever they are on the spectrum. They can teach your child to produce sounds, improve articulation, put together a proper sentence, and the like. They can also help children who struggle with back-and-forth conversational language. For example, if a child's main focus is trains, they can probably tell you about every type of train ever made, the year they were made, the railways they travel on and whether they were used for freight or public transportation. Although it's great for a child to take an interest in a particular subject, fixation on a topic makes it difficult to form relationships and establish reciprocal communication with others. A speech therapist can help redirect a child and teach more back-and-forth, conversational language.

Some children with ASD will speak in high tones or use unusual voices. Some children will only echo what the people around them say (echolalia). Others may be able to speak but need help initiating conversations and learning proper social etiquette. The goal is always to improve communication skills, and a therapist can help your child learn those skills.

When David started speech therapy, he was two years old and nonverbal. The goal of speech therapy for us was to increase communication and we did that by teaching him sign language. He only signed a few words such as *more, eat, drink,* and *I love you.* Let me digress for a moment and share a pivotal moment in his communication development. I remember praying, night after night, "Dear God, please, please let him say he loves me. That's all I ask. I need something to hope for, a sign he is in there. Please, God, let him tell me he loves me." One night, when David was four, I sat by his bed crying my eyes out. I said, "Please tell me you love me, David. Mommy needs it. It's this sign, and I showed him the *I love you* sign he'd learned from his therapist, remember? Please tell me you love me, David. I need it." I woke up, he was sleeping in his fire truck bed which was at the foot of my bed and saw that he was staring right at me. He saw my eyes open and immediately signed "I love you." It was so moving. It gave me the motivation to keep pushing, and to keep looking for ways to help him communicate. That moment was very affirming for me. I knew that he was in there, trying to get out, and it was my job to make sure that happened.

Getting back to the subject, yes, sign language is an option for nonverbal kids. In addition, I feel that children with ASD should be taught to read as early as possible. I have a video for teaching children to read which can be accessed on my Facebook page.[3] Once a child can read, they can move on to alternative means of communication with an iPad, computer, word cards, or even writing their needs.

If a child is not taught to read, they can use *Picture Exchange Communication System* (PECS) or another type of "talker" which allows the child to communicate using pictures and simple sentences. PECS picture images can be found easily online. Whichever method you choose, the most important thing is that your child be able to communicate their needs. What if they have an earache? What if they have a cavity? What if something happened at day care or school? They have to be able to communicate basic needs and articulate if they are being mistreated.

It's really important to know how nonverbal people with autism feel about their world. Timothy Ryan is an adult with autism, he uses the Rapid Prompt Method to write and communicate with the people around him. In a journal entry posted on Age of Autism, he wrote about his experience at

Disneyland and on the airplane ride home: His comments, cited below are from his journal:

> The Disney Park was hot, steamy, muggy, and smelly. My family and I were waiting for the Splash Mountain ride. I felt sick. My body was on fire from the inside out. My head was going to explode. I couldn't talk and describe the agony.[4]

The purpose of speech therapy isn't always to teach the child to speak; sometimes the goal is for the therapist is to find the right device or program that will enable the child to communicate that they are feeling "agony." Keep in mind, Timothy's description of being "on fire" is very similar to how many children with autism explain sensory overload.

Timothy goes on to describe the plane ride home:

> The airplane was cramped, dirty, noisy, and uncomfortable. Cigarette smoke lingered in the cabin. I became sick, nauseous, and disoriented. Passengers were staring at me with ugly faces. It felt like I was on display at the museum. Dad was aware of my discomfort due to relentless pummeling from my fists. Mom was mortified by my seemingly irrational behavior.[5]

You see, most of the so-called bad behavior we see from our kids with autism is really just an inability to effectively communicate. They aren't bad, they are overwhelmed, and people staring at them and judging their behavior only adds to the negative behavior:

> I felt as if my body was breaking down like an old used car. It hurt to breathe, think, talk, and be around people. People make it impossible for me to interact. They speak too rapidly and don't wait

for me to respond. If only they would notice how I am trying to fit in and be more typical. It would help if people made an effort to get to know me. I am suffering from an illness that robs me from establishing relationships. I can feel rejection. It hurts to see others move forward while I remain trapped in my inner world. It is not my choice to be disabled and dependent upon people.[6]

Timothy is no different from any other nonverbal person on the spectrum and is absolutely the same inside as the rest of us. How would you feel if you were in pain, if people were staring at you, and if you knew that the police could detain you, all the while being incapable of controlling your actions? It would be horrifying. Our kids aren't bad, they aren't trying to ruin our day, they are overwhelmed and need a way to communicate their needs.

There are many avenues to pursue for communication. Timothy's mother chose the Rapid Prompt Method, but you can decide which method will work best for your child. I'll leave you with one last glimpse of life with nonverbal autism:

> He has spelled for us that he has been hurt by the way others have treated him over the years. One incident that stands out for him was when he was 6 and the director of a special education school he attended told the principal of the school that he was unteachable—right in front of him. He has spelled for us that he has understood everything that has ever been said around or to him.[7]

Our kids with autism may be understanding absolutely everything that is said around them. Our job, with the help of a speech therapist, is to give them the tools they need to communicate. I can't imagine living through 17 years of childhood and adolescence not being able to speak. It's heartbreaking.

I'll try to keep the other therapy summaries shorter, but I feel that communication, verbal or otherwise, is an absolute right and necessity. Because this topic is so complex, I'll refer you to my favorite autism organization for more information: TACA has resources under "Helping Nonverbal Kids to Communicate" with information and links on augmentative devices, facilitated communication, keyboarding, and the like.[8]

Occupational therapy

Occupational therapy is a lifesaver for children who struggle with fine and gross motor skills. When David started occupational therapy (OT), he was two years old. Five therapists quit, three were asked to leave, most of them lasting no more than two sessions with him. He would not respond to their requests, wouldn't sit through a therapy session, and he hit, kicked, bit or spit on most of them. It wasn't until we found Cindy that he was able to make progress. Cindy started with David when he was four (technically, she's an occupational therapy assistant). It took her two years just to get him to write his own name. Two years! She was hit, kicked, and screamed at, yet she refused to give up on him. She cares about his future and his well-being. This is the type of OT you need. It has to be someone who is committed to the betterment of your child's future.

The primary function of OT is to teach skills needed in the real world. An OT can help with handwriting (it took six months just to get David to *hold* a pencil), using scissors, eating, drinking, hand washing, riding a bike, sensory processing, social skills, and appropriate play skills. The intent of OT is to improve the quality of life for your child by teaching motor skills which are essential to daily life. An OT can help with things that are very difficult for a parent to teach.

Until recently David had a lot of sensory issues with eating. I think some textures triggered a sensory response and he would either gag or refuse to try new foods. Because he has so many food allergies, I needed to expand his diet to include foods he had a sensory response to. Cindy thought that allowing him to use an electric toothbrush would help to desensitize his mouth. I bought a couple cheap electric toothbrushes for $5 apiece at Target. It took a while, but eventually he got used to them. After a couple months of using the electric toothbrush, he started trying new foods, including mashed potatoes and scrambled eggs! I thought I'd never see the day.

Another issue we had was him dressing himself. David hated buttons, tying his shoes, and using zippers. Cindy was well equipped to address these activities of daily living. She brought in a board that had a zipper on it and made it a game. She had another board that had a picture of a shoe and real shoelaces stapled to it. They practiced, for a year, tying the string on the board until David was ready to apply that skill to his own shoes. OT can help with fine motor skills and a good OT can change the life of a child. If at first you don't succeed (at finding an awesome therapist), try, and try again.

Applied Behavioral Analysis (ABA)

ABA is based on B. F. Skinner's principles of conditioning. In a nutshell, positive behaviors are rewarded, and negative behaviors are not. A child's behaviors are analyzed, and strategies are implemented based on the child's needs. Parents work with the ABA therapist to set target goals and behaviors. This can be anything from appropriate social behavior to something as routine as crossing the street safely. The Autism Research Institute was one of the first autism organizations to recommend ABA therapy for children on the spectrum. It modifies behavior by reinforcing the desired behavior.

I didn't have the money for ABA when David was little, but I did my own version of it at home. When he went potty in the potty, I gave him a piece of candy. If he picked up his toys or threw something away in the trash, I gave him a piece of candy then too. I used ABA to get him to sit at the table for dinner (this took six months) as well as for daily routines such as getting his coat on and letting me tie his shoes. I used positive reinforcement on a daily basis. I would say, "great job" and give him a high-five when he sat down to let me tie his shoes (for example). His little face would light up. Positive reinforcement is key for children with autism. Oftentimes our kids hear what they're doing wrong more than they hear what they are doing right. Positive reinforcement is very powerful. Sometimes that might be a reward like a piece of candy or a sticker. The goal is to always be reinforcing the desired behavior with an external reward (like candy, stickers, high-fives, etc.).

I gradually phased out the candy as a way to reinforce a desired behavior, over the course of three months, and replaced it with a little toy, compliment, or a high-five. My version of ABA helped David tremendously and ABA as a whole has been very successful at modifying behavior in many children with autism. If you have the opportunity to enroll your child in a good ABA program, I would recommend doing so. Appropriate behavior, peer interactions, safety skills, and the like are often skills that must be taught to our kids. ABA will help your child to achieve the goals that you feel are most important. It's best to start ABA at a very young age, but if you are not able to hire a professional right away, you can apply the basic principles at home.

Relationship Development Intervention

Relationship Development Intervention (RDI) is founded on the idea that you must form a relationship with a child in order to teach him or her new skills. I love the idea of RDI because it helps parents establish a relationship and bond with their child. For some families that bond comes naturally, but for many others it needs to be taught. RDI will give parents the skills they need to teach their child empathy, play skills, and other important social skills. RDI can be taught by a therapist but should always be reinforced in the home.

The concept of RDI is quite brilliant. Kids with autism often don't automatically understand social skills and need to be taught how to interact and how to play with others. RDI is effective because it gives parents skills and strategies to get their child to interact with family members in a safe environment. Once social skills are taught at home, our kids can apply these skills in school or in social settings.

RDI is a behavior therapy, and many ABA therapists have experience with RDI and can develop a treatment plan that includes both principles. Insurance and Medicaid waivers vary state to state, but many insurance plans will cover some form of RDI. Again, when David was little, my insurance company covered very little in the way of autism-related therapies, so I was forced to learn RDI on my own and develop my own treatment plan for him. If you cannot get this therapy covered, you can always take the core principles and apply them at home.

Floortime

Floortime is fantastic. It teaches parents and caregivers to meet the child where they are developmentally. Floortime encourages parents to enter their child's world and help them develop goals based on their child's interests. This therapy is centered around the child with autism and the parents learn to expand on the child's skill set.

If your child loves to line up their cars, get down on the floor and line up cars with him until he notices you are parallel playing with them. If your child is staring at the ceiling fan, you stare at the ceiling fan too. It comes down to engaging with your child and realizing that their behaviors aren't wrong: They line cars up or stare at ceiling fans because it brings them joy and helps them feel centered. When we learn to fully participate in our child's favorite activities, we build bonds and develop a relationship that allows us to teach them where they are developmentally. Floortime shows our kids that we appreciate them as they are. Like most of us, our kids want acceptance and love from those around them. Until they feel that unconditional love and acceptance, it is very difficult to teach them academics or life skills.

Once you have bonded with your child by engaging in activities they like, you can start to help them build new skills. If your child wants you to push them on a swing (for example) they will learn to communicate their desire through sign language, a hand gesture or verbal request. When we bond with our kids, we learn about their interests. When we know what they are interested in, we can use that to motivate them and teach social skills.

Son-Rise

Son-Rise is an interesting approach to therapy. I applied the core principles of Son-Rise at home with David when he was little. A friend of mine went to a Son-Rise seminar and spent several days learning about this therapeutic approach. What she taught me helped David develop both academic and social skills.

The most helpful advice she gave me was about the principle of *joining*. Joining means to join your child in his preferred activities. For example, David used to spin and flap his hands for hours every day. After I learned about joining, I would stand in his line of sight and spin when he spun and flap my hands when he flapped his hands. After some time, he actually started looking at me again! One day he was jumping, spinning and hand flapping. I mimicked him for probably thirty minutes, and then we had a breakthrough: He stopped, smiled at me, and laughed! He interacted with me for the first time in years! It was glorious!

The basic idea is to enter their world because, in many cases, they will not be inclined to enter your world. Once I bonded with David, I was able to teach him to read and do math. Because I applied the principle of joining at home, I was able to teach him academics. I believe that one of the reasons David is on track academically is because I applied the core principles of Son-Rise all those years ago.

If you are able to attend a Son-Rise seminar, great! If not, they have resources online and books available for purchase as well.[9]

Physical therapy

Although David did not need physical therapy (PT), I realize some of our kids struggle with gross motor skills. Gross motor skills include things like crawling, running, swimming, and overall coordination. If your child needs help enhancing gross motor skills, it would probably be beneficial to seek out a physical therapist.

Physical therapists can help pinpoint areas of concern such as low muscle tone, limited range of motion, poor endurance, and overall strength. A physical therapist will work on setting goals to increase gross motor skills and will likely give you a list of exercises that your child can do at home. A physical therapist can also establish whether your child will benefit from adaptive equipment like a ramp (instead of stairs to enter the home), leg braces, or wheelchairs. The goal of PT is to enhance gross motor skills, as opposed to OT which focuses more on fine motor skills. If you feel your child has physical delays, be sure to ask the diagnosing physician for a referral to either PT, OT, or both. If no such recommendations are made at the time of diagnosis, your child's school may request an evaluation of their own to ensure OT and PT are included at school. Keep in mind, if you feel a particular therapy will benefit your child, most insurance companies will approve therapy if they have a written note from the pediatrician's office.

Pivotal Response Training

Pivotal Response Training (PRT) is a therapy method used to increase speech and social behavior skills. I am not a therapist; I'm a mom. I see things from a mother's perspective. I learned about PRT from one of David's brilliant therapists. This therapist is a *Board Certified Behavior Analyst* (BCBA), and he changed our lives. What makes David's BCBA so effective is his passion for helping kids who have autism. Dedicated therapists do so much more for our kids than people who are just showing up for a paycheck.

David's therapist has gotten him to speak in full sentences, answer questions in a full sentence, and to participate in age-appropriate activities such as taking turns playing video games and engaging in back-and-forth conversations. The BCBA uses many techniques to get David to communicate. One thing that has been particularly helpful is the communication chart they use during therapy. The BCBA writes down numbers, 1, 2, 3, 4, and 5, and David writes down five things he'd like to talk about. The BCBA started with one topic and has increased it to five topics. For every topic David chooses (usually things like Mario Bros., YouTube videos, or music), he must say two sentences about it. Each time David says a sentence, he gets a check mark. If he says two sentences for each topic, he can choose an activity to do for a few minutes. The BCBA says two sentences for each topic as well and they practice various responses David can give like, "I like that too," or "Tell me more." This simple chart has been hugely impactful in David's language development.

A good BCBA will address social skills, conversational

language, safety skills, and overall behavior. When PRT is included into the therapy regimen, it addresses a number of core issues. PRT is modeled on the following protocols:

1. The instruction has to be clear, appropriate to the task, uninterrupted, and the child has to be attending to the therapist or task;
2. Maintenance tasks need to be interspersed frequently;
3. Multiple cues need to be presented if appropriate for the child's developmental level;
4. The child needs to be given a significant role in choosing the stimulus item(s);
5. Rewards need to be immediate, contingent, uninterrupted, and effective;
6. Direct reinforcers need to be used the majority of the time; and
7. Rewards need to be contingent on response attempts.[10]

Hippotherapy

No, it is not a typo, and no, it has nothing to do with hippopotamuses. It is horseback riding therapy. I wish I could say David had experienced hippotherapy. We tried horseback riding when he was about five but he got red, itchy eyes and started sneezing like crazy. He has tried a couple times since then and although he has had a very minimal allergic response (itchy eyes), I was reluctant to sign him up for long-term hippotherapy until his allergies improved.

I have heard so many wonderful things about hippotherapy for kids with autism. Hippotherapy benefits children with autism because they can connect with a living being and not have the pressure of having to speak and socialize. It can also help a child gain physical strength and can build up core muscles.

Hippotherapy is covered by some Medicaid waivers and some insurance plans. If your state's waiver does not cover it, you can request funding through your disability resource center. If your particular insurance company does not cover this therapy, remember you can always write a letter of medical necessity. This is probably one of my favorite therapies because it is a joyous experience for our kids. Most therapies are not especially fun for them, and I like that hippotherapy is something they can enjoy. Enjoying therapy is important; when the goal is to learn and develop new skills, the process should be fun. Hippotherapy gets them outside in the fresh air and builds core muscles; it's a win-win.

If you aren't sure how your child would respond to this therapy, you can try reaching out to a local hippotherapy center and ask to bring your child in for a day or two to see how they respond to horses.

Social Thinking

Social Thinking is awesome! One of the biggest challenges our kids face is learning how to socialize, and Social Thinking (let's call it ST for short) helps address social skills in a very unique and powerful way. Using ST, our kids are taught to initiate conversations, which for many seem difficult, if not impossible. Verbal and nonverbal children can benefit from ST because initiation can begin whether the child is verbal or not.

Children learn basic social skills at a very young age. Typically, children learn to read facial expressions, body language, and turn taking while playing with other children and interacting with family. Our kids are expected to sit in a classroom and focus, interact with peers and siblings, and respond to social cues in a typical manner despite not having developed these critical skills. For example, young children will generally learn to interpret another person's body language, emotions, and even intentions. If our children don't automatically acquire these skills, they must be taught social thinking in a structured manner. The social thinking behaviors a child would usually learn on the playground such as taking turns, group participation, self-regulation, and safety need to be modeled.

In her video ST founder Michelle Garcia Winner explains that imagination is a key factor in learning. When we think about the social mind, we often think about having fun, meeting new people, and participating in group activities. What we as parents and educators often miss is the importance of imagination pertaining to academic learning. Children with autism often lack imaginative play skills and that impacts learning for a variety of reasons. Let's say your child's teacher is reading a book about sailing the ocean; a child's imagination should provide mental images of water, dolphins, blue sky, rain. If a child lacks that imagination piece, sitting through a story about sailing the ocean becomes boring and lacks meaning. If the child is then expected to retell the story, there is a lack of associated vocabulary to express the details and related images. Imagination is also required to explain an idea; we must first imagine before we can explain the idea in detail.

Social thinking is not inherent in all people with autism. If your child struggles with this, ST can help with social behavior—which extends to learning, classroom behavior, work habits and relationships. Social thinking "affects the person's social skills, perspective taking, self-awareness, self-regulation, critical thinking, social problem solving, play skills, reading comprehension, written expression, ability to learn and work in a group, organizational skills, etc." "Only as individuals gain awareness of their own thoughts, emotions, and intentions can they become increasingly aware of the thoughts, emotions, intentions, and actions of others."[11] ST incorporates ideas from Theory of Mind which can be beneficial to our kids as well. Theory of Mind is the understanding that one's thoughts and mental states are one's own and different from those of others. People with autism often struggle to relate to others because they don't always realize that others think differently than they do. This is an abstract concept to some people on the spectrum and difficult to grasp; therefore, it has to be taught.

This particular intervention has had a tremendous impact on David and his ability to communicate, retell stories, and learn in a general education classroom. When I was interviewing new BCBAs for David, I was struck by one therapist in particular. He mentioned something called "head in group, head not in group," which I had not heard of. This lesson helps the child with autism to learn social skills in a group setting with a tangible model. The children at the table all have a Play-Doh person. If the child with autism is not listening or is turned in the other direction, the little Play-Doh person is either removed from the group or the head is removed to indicate that their mind is not in the group. It is a meaningful way (without reprimanding them) to show them what it looks like to physically be withdrawn from the group's activities. It gives them a visual as to what looking away or turning away feels like to their friends. When the BCBA told me about this concept, I thought to myself, *This is our guy.* As I have stated previously, therapy is important, but the therapist is key. A good, highly qualified therapist will have a variety of teaching methods to help your child gain skills. Our therapist incorporates ST into David's program but also uses other behavior-based interventions to help him make gains.

The ST website is very informative, and a parent can learn a ton about this intervention online if they can't afford therapy immediately. Michelle Garcia Winner has books and posters for sale and articles parents can access for free or at a minimal cost. Although I recommend that a trained professional work with your child, if that is not in the cards right now, her website provides plenty of resources for parents on a budget.

Music therapy

According to The American Music Therapy Association, music therapy will address "behavioral, social, psychological, communicative, physical, sensory motor, and/or cognitive functioning. Because music therapy is a powerful and non-threatening medium, unique outcomes are possible."[12]

To me, music therapy makes sense because it gives a child the opportunity to engage in something they may actually *want* to do. David loves music. He listens to The Beatles often, but more than anything he *loves* to listen to Adele. But I mean, he *LOVES* Adele, with a passion. He listens to "Hello" about fifty times a day if not more. If Adele were played during music therapy, I can see how it would engage, motivate, and inspire him to learn.

It's logical to think that our kids would benefit from music therapy as it involves their interests and their choices. The American Music Therapy Association states:

> Music holds universal appeal. It provides a bridge in a non-threatening setting between people and/or between individuals and their environment, facilitating relationships, learning, self-expression, and communication. Music captures and helps maintain attention.[13]

Rapid Prompt Method (RPM)

I don't know that RPM is considered a therapy as much as it is an intervention—designed to help our children build communication and academic skills. RPM was developed by autism mama Soma Mukhopadhyay. Soma holds advanced degrees in neuroscience but had no formal training in autism. She developed her own method for teaching her son Tito academics by having him point to letters and numbers and physically guide him in learning new tasks such as riding a bike.

By the time Tito was six, he could write independently, and by age eleven, he was evaluated by the National Autistic Society (UK) and determined to be gifted. Soma's methods are effective because they emphasize the importance of education and finding a way to teach our kids despite their behaviors. Tito, like many children with autism, could not learn in a traditional educational setting, and Soma learned that with the right support and tools her child could excel in academics.

Over the years, I have noticed that when a child with autism has negative behaviors, schools tend to focus on behavior interventions and learning becomes secondary. RPM takes a different approach, "Despite behaviors, the academic focus of every RPM lesson is designed to activate the reasoning part of the brain so that the student becomes distracted by and engaged in learning."[14] RPM factors autistic behaviors into their program and has found a way to teach our kids, even while they are having behaviors. It's really quite brilliant.

RPM stays true to its name. It is a rapid approach to learning. To me, it makes sense because our kids are often very smart, but they are easily distracted and may lose interest easily. RPM moves so quickly, they have little time for distractions or daydreaming. If a child has no language, RPM teaches him or her to communicate by pointing to letters and, eventually, written words. It moves rapidly and keeps the child engaged while stimulating parts of the brain associated with learning.

RPM is not a therapy per se; it is more of an intervention parents can use if their child is struggling with learning and/or communicating. In many cases, the saying "necessity is the mother of invention" applies to parenting a child with autism. Oftentimes, the professionals around us are at a loss as how to help our children make gains. RPM can change how your child learns and communicates. There are plenty of free or reasonably priced resources online to help you get started!

Emotional Freedom Technique
(EFT or "Tapping")

Is tapping a traditional therapy for autism? No. However, when we reach a point where traditional, therapy methods are not helping our child make progress, we often start to think outside the box. The Tapping Solution (EFT as practiced by Nicholas Ortner and described in his book and documentary films of the same name) was shown to me by a friend and autism mama who believed it helped her child's behaviors decrease.

Tapping is explained as providing:

> ...relief from chronic pain, emotional problems, disorders, addictions, phobias, post-traumatic stress disorder, and physical diseases. While Tapping is newly set to revolutionize the field of health and wellness, the healing concepts that it's based upon have been in practice in Eastern medicine for over 5,000 years.[15]

This method is intended to help our kids release the emotional stress they feel. Our kids are often treated differently by teachers, by relatives, and by their peers. They spend most of their childhood in therapy, and many of our kids have painful, underlying medical conditions. When you look at the cumulative effect of emotional and physical pain, it makes sense that our kids need a way to release these pent-up emotions.[16]

EFT is not something every parent would try, but for parents who are open to Eastern medicine and unconventional methods of healing, it is worth a try. Tapping uses acupressure points and is meant to help release negative emotions such as anxiety and fear. If a child has high anxiety, the anxiety can be difficult to treat: all medications aimed at lowering anxiety have drawbacks, and it can be difficult to get children with sensory issues to take supplements. The Tapping Solution is designed to help decrease anxiety and post-traumatic stress disorders (PTSD).

Although I am not opposed to medication in all cases, I know that there are no behavior meds approved for autism. Doctors can make an educated guess as to which medications to prescribe, but each child's biochemistry is different. It's impossible to know how a child will react to any given prescribed medication. I know of several children with autism who were put on behavior meds only to have their behaviors increase. When the behaviors increased, they were put on more meds to counteract the effects of the first medication. When I caved and put David on a behavior med, he became lethargic and slept most of the day, which in my opinion was not much of a solution. I didn't want him to be a tiny zombie; I wanted his negative behaviors to decrease.

The point is I understand why we reach out to doctors for help with behavior. Behaviors associated with autism can be very difficult to deal with. I know that some parents report their child benefited from medication, and in some cases, it may help decrease behaviors. In my mind, addressing the underlying medical causes of the behavior and helping the child release pent-up emotions is a part of the equation. We are all doing the best we can. If you as a parent feel medication is necessary, that is your choice. If you are opposed to medication, you should know there are options, and EFT may help your child release negative emotions and feel centered. There are no negative side effects, and it can't hurt to try it.

Energy healing

Energy healing is fairly new to me, but as I gather it is clearing energy blockage in the body. Anne M. Evans is a microbiologist who healed her daughter's autism via energy healing. Anne's assertion is that once the toxic load in the body has decreased, symptoms of autism will decrease as well. While there are many forms of energy healing, Anne's approach incorporates *Nambudripad's Allergy Elimination Technique (NAET)*. NAET uses acupressure to correct allergy symptoms, relieve the body of stagnation, and allow toxins to flow from the body, which then allows energy to flow freely.

Anne has written a book called *Beating Autism* and offers coaching to families affected by autism. Her website also provides links to scientific research and services provided.[17]

Although I am new to this idea, I am always open to listening to parents who have recovered their child. Anne's approach is different from standard autism treatments. Her daughter has lost the diagnosis of autism and is currently in college. Conventional or not, this is worth looking into if you are looking for noninvasive methods of treatment.

KNOW THAT YOU CAN CHANGE DIRECTION AT ANY TIME

Therapy can be tricky. When our journey began, I thought that I needed to drive David an hour across town for OT, even though I had the option of having an in-home OT. I felt obligated to stick with therapists who weren't effective because I didn't want to hurt anyone's feelings.

As time went on I became more assertive and gained the courage to set boundaries. When I saw that a therapy was not helping him or the particular therapist was not able to meet his needs, I moved on. Sometimes asserting ourselves can be uncomfortable and awkward, but in the end it may be necessary to our child's development.

The purpose of therapy is to help our kids make gains. After giving it a fair chance, if a particular therapy is not helping, it is okay to move on to a different type of therapy. If, for example, you have tried behavior therapy for six months but notice your child is suffering from sensory overload and can't sit through therapy, maybe hire an OT who can work with the behavior therapist to address sensory sensitivities. If your child has been in speech therapy for a year and can now verbalize his or her needs but can't initiate conversations, maybe add behavior therapy to the regimen.

Somewhere along the way I learned to give suggestions to David's therapists without being critical or negative; the book, *How to Win Friends and Influence People*, by Dale Carnegie, helped me with this. I learned the importance of his school therapists and in-home therapists being on the same page. I learned that therapy is most effective if reinforced at home.

In time you will find therapies that work well for your child. David seemed to benefit most from the traditional therapies for autism such as OT, speech, and behavior therapy. However, as I mentioned, I added in my own version of Son-Rise to complement the therapies he was receiving. Your child may benefit from music and hippotherapy, for example. You know your child best, and because you are the expert on your child, you should feel empowered to choose or abstain from any given therapy. You should always have a voice in their treatment and therapy plans.

As the poem so beautifully reminds us, we are blessed to be a part of their lives, "Blessed are you who never bid us to 'hurry up' and more blessed are you who do not snatch our tasks from our hands and do them for us, for often we need time rather than help."

Our kids can accomplish great things with time, patience, biomedical interventions, and the right therapies. Therapy can change the course of a child's life. In time you will find the right therapists. And for those of you who have nonverbal children, please know that there are ways to help your child communicate. My deepest desire was to hear David tell me he loved me, and just last week he lay down with me and said, "I love you so, so much, Mother. You are the best mother."

Never give up!

NOTES FOR CHAPTER 5

6

EDUCATION

Every student can learn, just not on the same day, or in the same way.

—George Evans[1]

EDUCATION IS A LEGAL right in the United States. Special education, for which many of our children qualify, is a different avenue for children to access curricula and a quality public education. The goal for all students is to receive a well-rounded education which includes a variety of subjects. Not all of our kids are going to fit the traditional educational model, but they certainly can learn and, with a proper education, can achieve the goals they set for themselves or we set for them. Whether their goal is to be a mechanic, a computer programmer, or a teacher or to work with animals at a shelter, their goals can be realized and nurtured though special education services.

Special education services are protected by the *Americans with Disabilities Act* (ADA) and the *Individuals with Disabilities Education Act* (IDEA), which falls under the umbrella of the ADA. Learning how to make the most of your child's *individualized education plan* (IEP) requires basic knowledge of the ADA and the IDEA and how to successfully negotiate (without crying, yelling, or jumping across the table) during IEP meetings.

It took me years to learn the ADA and IDEA, and I certainly don't want you to have to learn the system from scratch as I did. The most important thing a parent can do to facilitate their child's education is to be empowered. The best way to empower yourself is to know special education law and, therefore, your child's legal rights under IDEA. I will include books and wonderful resources for you in this chapter but will also provide you with the information you need to know to ensure your child receives a quality public education.

David has been in exceptional public school programs with people who loved, understood, and educated him. On the other hand, he has also been in terrible programs where he was left on a school bus for hours in the cold and was with people who spent more time texting in the classroom than they did educating him. We have had both good and bad experiences at school; over time I have learned to navigate the system successfully and have found legal avenues to hold schools and individuals accountable when David's legal rights have been violated.

Learning special education law is necessary for most parents of children with autism because, let's face it, not every teacher, teacher's aide, or administrator has received quality autism education and training. I have sat in meetings with administrators (school principals and vice-principals) who seem to have never read IDEA or know our kids' legal rights. This is a common scenario. Sometimes we end up in meetings with people who simply don't know special education law well enough to protect our child's rights and, therefore, cannot provide a quality education for a child with an IEP. Then there are scenarios where school-district personnel, usually special education directors and team members know the law but stand in opposition to the best interest of the child and the parents' wishes. Whatever the situation may be, knowing your child's rights will allow you to negotiate effectively with special education teams and

IEP teams and will give you the tools needed to hold school districts accountable if they fail to meet your child's educational needs.

Unfortunately, voters often fail to support school districts with tax money. Given the fact that one in thirty-six boys now has autism, the need for funding has never been greater. There may be occasions when school districts have adequate resources and still fail to meet our kids' needs, but in most cases school districts cannot begin to meet the needs of kids with autism without the financial support of taxpayers. School districts are required by federal law to accommodate our children. Those in-school accommodations include additional teachers' aides for classroom support, occupational therapy, speech therapy, physical therapy, mental health services, classroom support, and transportation. If funding is not supported for these vital services, schools can only provide a fraction of what is required of them by law.

The best way to handle a problem is to be proactive. As parents of children with autism, we are our children's voices. We need to speak to our legislators, neighbors, and family members to increase autism awareness as well as funding in our schools. Raising David has taught me that anything is possible. Persistence has won me more battles than I can recall, and it will do the same for you. Whether the issue you face is small or enormous, persistence combined with knowledge of facts and belief in yourself can move mountains.

This chapter will empower you to be your child's advocate. It will teach you commonly used acronyms, how to prepare your child for the classroom, how to negotiate an effective IEP, and how to navigate conflict resolution. The list of things to do for this chapter can change your child's educational experience. So, let's get to it.

- Empower yourself by learning your child's legal rights
- Learn the essential acronyms for IEP meetings
- Prepare your child for academic success
- Prepare for the IEP
- Learn how to resolve educational conflict

EMPOWER YOURSELF BY LEARNING YOUR CHILD'S LEGAL RIGHTS

Raising a child with autism impacts parents in a variety of ways; for several years, I felt that my strength had diminished. The stares from people in public chipped away at my power. I felt drained by friends, family members—and even strangers—with their constant inquisitions: "What is wrong with him?" "How do you stop the screaming?" "Why is he hitting himself?" "Can't you stop it?" I felt drained because I am his mom. I was supposed to know how to help my son and I didn't. The feeling of powerlessness as his mother changed who I was as a person. It would be years until I got my strength back and felt empowered again.

How did I get my power back? I took it back.

Let's start at the beginning. When David was in an autism-centered program for preschool, it was wonderful. The teachers and staff were angels on Earth. They were patient, kind and invested in each one of their students. David's autism was severe, and they did everything under the sun to help support and educate him. I assumed the transition to kindergarten would be easy and that the staff at his new school would be just as kind and professional as his preschool. Boy was I in for a rude awakening.

We had David's transition meeting, a meeting you have when transitioning from one school to another, at the end of his last year of preschool. The meeting was held at what would be his new elementary school. When I saw the classroom and newly stocked sensory room, I was blown away! It was a great set-up for my son. The sensory room was right next door to the classroom and was there to provide the kids a sensory break if they were overstimulated and needed to regroup. The classroom and sensory room were a selling point for me and I agreed to place David in this particular school with its autism-centered program because it appeared to have the right supports in place to meet my son's needs.

When I arrived at David's new school, I was so excited! I had taken pictures of his new classrooms and teachers so that he was mentally prepared for his new environment. When I walked in the building with his tiny backpack and bags of school supplies, I was met by a secretary who asked, "Which classroom are you looking for?" I replied, "The ASD room, but I know where it is, thank you. I'll take him down there." She responded, "Well, they moved the ASD kids outside. You need to take him to the temporary buildings." Shocked, I responded, "Do you mean the buildings right by the street? He will run in the street. I spent the entire summer showing him pictures of his classrooms. He is going to have a melt-down if I take him to those buildings." Her response was, "That is up to the principal. Take it up with her."

And so it began. My ascent from bewildered, broken-down autism mom to fierce and powerful advocate for my son began that day. I knew that placing these kids near a street would be trouble and that my son's life would be in jeopardy due to this ill-planned physical placement. I spoke to the principal who was not interested in anything I had to say. I spoke to the district's special education team who were not interested in moving the kids back into the main building.

For the next several months, I pleaded with the principal and special education directors to move the kids back into the school. I was met with hostility and scoffs, and before long they all stopped returning my phone calls. I tried my best to be pleasant and understanding, but it got me nowhere.

Around this time I attended an informational meeting on IEPs at the Autism Society of Colorado. At this meeting they spoke about special education law and provided us all with a book called *The Everyday Guide to Special Education Law* by Randy Chapman.[2] I went home and started to read. I also started doing my own research on IDEA.

As it turns out, it is illegal to physically separate children with disabilities from their peers; doing so can be considered discrimination. I, again, called the principal and special education directors and explained that this placement was not legal and that they needed to move the kids' classrooms back into the building. I also informed them that a child with autism almost ran in front of a car, and I had to run out and pull him back onto the curb. Had I not been there at that exact moment, the child (who had no safety-awareness skills) would have been hit by a car. They did not return my calls, so guess what I did? I called my local news station and explained that children with autism were being segregated and that the district was not in compliance with federal law; 9News here in Colorado came out and reported on the story. Sure enough, they moved the autism program back into the school the next day.

Although I try to always be polite and kind, there are people in this world who do not respond to courtesy and kindness. There are circumstances which require us to be bold and have courage, even if we don't feel up to it. The principal at David's elementary school and the district personnel I contacted were not interested in addressing their violation of federal law even though I gave them several opportunities to do so. As much as I wanted everyone at his school to like me, I realized that I was going to have to make people uncomfortable in order to do what was right for my son.

I was empowered enough to call the news because I knew my son's legal rights under IDEA. I learned about special education law from a law book a friend of mine gave me and the book mentioned above. I take *The Everyday Guide* with me to every IEP meeting and put it on the table for everyone to see. If something comes up and I need to reference the law, I have my handy book right there to curb any shenanigans. You do not have to be an expert on special education law to successfully negotiate an IEP; knowing even the basics of special education law can go a long way.

In addition to *The Everyday Guide*, I really like Wrightslaw. Wrightslaw has a website with helpful tips and up-to-date information on special education law.[3] They have a blog, books for sale, a "game plan for new parents," flyers and case law.

The best way to empower yourself is knowledge. Learning special education law does not mean you have to be a lawyer or advocate, it simply means knowing your child's legal rights under IDEA. It can also mean learning the lingo commonly used in IEP meetings, which brings me to my next point, learning the most commonly uses acronyms for IEP meetings.

LEARN THE ESSENTIAL ACRONYMS FOR IEP MEETINGS

When I went to David's transition meeting for kindergarten, I was so confused I literally didn't understand what the IEP team was saying. I wasn't even very clear on what an IEP was. They were saying things like, "The SLP will put his evaluation in his Cumulative Record. Your CCB sent us his evaluations, and we think he'd benefit from OT and SLP, but doesn't require PT. He qualifies for ASD programming, and that gives us the option of moving forward with an evaluation for AAC. Do you agree?" I remember sitting there thinking, *Am I supposed to know this? Do all autism moms know this lingo?* It was almost embarrassing. I wanted my son to have the best education possible, and while I understood that I was part of that process, I felt overwhelmed and unable to keep up with the conversation.

Looking back, I realize *why* I was overwhelmed. I was overwhelmed because, like most parents, I didn't know the acronyms used during IEP meetings and I felt lost in the conversation. In order to feel like we are a part of the conversation and contributing to our child's IEP, we need to be able to follow along during these meetings. Below is a list of commonly used acronyms that will help you navigate IEP meetings successfully.

The most commonly used acronyms for special education are:

AAC – Assistive and Augmentative Communication

ABA – Applied Behavior Analysis

ABC – Autism Behavior Checklist

ABLLS – Assessment of Basic Language Skills test

ADA – Americans with Disabilities Act

ADOS – Autism Diagnostic Observation Scale

APD – Auditory Processing Disorder

The ARC (Formerly known as The Association for Retarded Citizens) – Resources and Community Support

AS – Asperger's Syndrome

AS – Autism Spectrum

ASA – Autism Society of America

ASD – Autism Spectrum Disorder

ASHA – American Speech & Hearing Association

ASL – American Sign Language

ASPEN – Asperger Syndrome Parent Education Network

Aspie – A person with Asperger's Syndrome

BBRS – Burks' Behavior Rating Scale

BCBA – Board Certified Behavior Analyst

BIP – Behavior Improvement (or Intervention) Plan

BSC – Behavioral Specialist Consultant

CARS – Center for Autism and Related Disorders
CHAT – Checklist for Autism in Toddlers
COTA – Certified Occupational Therapy Assistant
Cum – Cumulative Educational Records of File
DAS – Developmental Apraxia of Speech
DD – Department of Disabilities
DD – Developmental delay (or) disorder
DSM – Diagnostic Statistical Manual
DX – Diagnosis
EFD – Executive Functioning Disorder
EPSDT – Early Periodic Screening, Diagnosis and
   Treatment Program
ESE – Exceptional Student Education
ESL – English as a Second Language
FAPE – Free Appropriate Public Education
FC – Facilitated Communication
FERPA – Federal Educational Rights and Privacy
   Act
FOIA – Freedom of Information Act
GARS – Gilliam Autism Rating Scale
HFA – High Functioning Autism
HI – Hearing Impaired
HSLDA – Home School Legal Defense Association
IAES – Interim Alternative Educational Setting
IDEA – Individuals with Disabilities Education Act
   IDEA Part B – Educational Services (age 3–22)
   IDEA Part C – Educational Services (up to age 3)
IEP – Individualized Education Plan
IFSP – Individualized Family Service Plan
IME – Independent Medical Evaluation
IQ – Intelligence Quotient
LD – Learning Disability
LEA – Local Education Agency
LRE – Least Restrictive Environment
NT – Neurotypical
OCD –Obsessive Compulsive Disorder

OCR – Office of Civil Rights
ODD – Oppositional Defiance Disorder
OSEP – Office of Special Education Programs
OT – Occupational Therapist
OVR – Office of Vocational Rehabilitation
PANDAS – Pediatric Autoimmune Neurological
    Disorder Associated with Strep
PANS – Pediatric Acute-onset Neuropsychiatric
    Syndrome
PBS – Positive Behavior Support
PDD – Pervasive Developmental Disorder
PECS – Picture Exchange Communication System
PRT – Pivotal Response Training
RDI – Relationship Development Intervention
SI – Sensory Integration
SLP – Speech Language Pathologist
Sped – Special Education
TBI – Traumatic Brain Injury
TEACCH – Treatment and Education of Autistic and
    Communication Handicapped Children
TOPL – Test of Pragmatic Language
TS – Tourette's Syndrome
Voc-Ed – Vocational Education
VQ – Verbal IQ[4]

PREPARE YOUR CHILD FOR ACADEMIC SUCCESS

One of the most valuable experiences I had as a mother of a child with autism was working in a special education classroom for two years. I learned about PBS (*positive behavior support*), strategies for de-escalating a child who is upset and how to approach academics with special-needs kids. The classes I took while working for Denver Public Schools helped me in the classroom and as a mother.

In addition to the training I received, I was able to get real-life experience working with special-needs kids in a classroom setting. It is not an easy job, and had I not worked in a classroom, I would not understand how hard teachers and teachers' aides work. It is a low-paying, difficult job. The burnout rate for special education teachers is very high, with the average teacher lasting about seven years.

Having two perspectives, both that of a professional and of a parent, I realized that a school can only do so much. We, as parents, must be a part of our child's education and must support the school and teachers when we can. Yes, there are instances when the school and teachers fail to meet the needs of our kids due to a lack of knowledge or professionalism, but by and large most teachers and teachers' aides aren't in it for the money. They are there because they genuinely care about the well-being of their students. That being said, I think it's important for us to be a part of our child's school community.

Most of us don't have a lot of extra time, but volunteering even two or three times a year can really help the teacher, which in turn helps your child succeed. Volunteering also gives you the opportunity to get to know the school staff. Oftentimes the classroom teacher, aides, or speech therapist (for example) will ask you questions about your child and how to best meet their needs; Volunteering is tricky. We are entering a classroom with kids who will be distracted by our presence, so I try staying in the back of the classroom or outside the classroom, making copies or performing other teacher-directed support. Teachers need the extra set of hands, and in most cases your time will be greatly appreciated.

When David was little and nonverbal I knew he understood me and was capable of learning. I was also acutely aware of the fact that he didn't test well and that teachers would underestimate his intelligence based on his test scores and inability to communicate. I felt like it was my responsibility to teach him to read and understand addition and subtraction before he entered kindergarten.

Teaching a nonverbal child with autism to read is not exactly an easy thing to do. Working at an elementary school, I learned that there is a song that, for whatever reason, can help teach most children to read. I'm not sure why it works; I only know that it does work. A link to the video is on my Facebook page. You can either show your child the video I made, or you can make your own letter cards and sing the song that goes with the cards. It's basically a phonics song: A-a-apple, B-b-ball, C-c-cat, and D-d-doll, etc.[5] Once the child knows the letters phonetically, you will introduce letter cards and use them to make words. I started with two- and three-letter words like up, ox, cat, hat, and bat and spent about two months on just those. The goal is for them to learn the alphabet phonetically and gain confidence by learning to spell and read three-letter words. Once your child has mastered three-letter words, you can add four- and five-letter words that coincide with the song's phonetic sounds such as ants, pants, can't, bent, and spent when working on the "nt" sound, and so on and so forth.

Once your child has mastered two- and three-letter words, you can make word cards to help them communicate. You can make a card for eat, as an example, and practice spelling it together. The next time your child eats a meal, put the card for *eat* next to him or her and say the word aloud. You can explain to them that if they give you the card for eat it means they are hungry and you will give them something to eat. You will walk them through the process of communicating by associating word cards to actions.

The purpose of this song is to learn the fundamentals of reading. Once our kids can read, they can use word cards to communicate their needs and wants, which will decrease behaviors. In addition to decreased behaviors, our kids will have an academic skill the school can work with and build on. I don't think it's unusual for a parent to teach their child to read, especially when it comes to kids who have autism. Our kids often have a hard time in the classroom because without basic skills like reading and writing, they probably feel bored and out of place in school. Teaching a child with autism to read can take a few months or maybe even years, but the benefits will last a lifetime. It will open doors and avenues for communication.

After I taught David to read, I transitioned to math. Before he regressed into autism he knew his alphabet and numbers, and I knew he had retained at least some of that information. At the time, David, Aidan, and I shared a bedroom at my parents' house (so glamorous, right?), and I put number cards with little pictures up on the wall. The cards had a number and a corresponding picture, e.g., the number one and one apple, the number two and two apples, etc. I started with numbers one through ten. I would point to them and count to ten several times a day. David almost never looked up at me while I counted, but I figured he was listening and retaining what I said.

I bought a little addition game which started with the numbers one through ten; each number had a spot for a little toy airplane below it. Eventually David took notice and we would place the airplanes on the numbers until I felt he could really count to ten in his mind. We then moved on to addition, one airplane + two airplanes = three airplanes. He would place the airplanes on the pictures and add them himself. Eventually, he could do this on his own, and we were able to move on to subtraction using this method. David had bad days where he threw the airplanes and attempted to tear up the cards (same with the letter cards, but I anticipated that and had them laminated, ha!), and I would calmly put everything away and bring it back out when he was having a good day.

Once he grasped the basics of addition and subtraction, I moved on to Touch Math. Touch Math is a simple and brilliant concept: numbers on a page have dots on them which correspond with the number; one has one dot, two has two dots, etc. I would pretend I was doing touch math myself by pointing to the dots and counting them out loud. I did this for several weeks before David seemed interested and wanted to join me. I then, hand over hand, pointed to the dots and we learned the numbers that way. We quickly transitioned to adding the numbers together by counting the dots on each number. Touch Math has free or inexpensive resources on their website if this is something you want to pursue.[6]

In addition to my methods of teaching David to read and write, I found LeapFrog products extremely helpful. I bought David a LeapFrog keyboard he could plug into the TV and use to play learning games. The refrigerator magnets helped him with spelling. He also had a minor obsession with Starfall. Starfall is a website that has reading and math games that kids love. David played Starfall at school and at home for several years, and I truly believe it helped him develop core reading and math skills. Starfall is designed in a way that makes learning fun and interactive. It's a great learning tool for kids who love technology.[7]

The purpose of teaching our kids to read and do basic math is simple: We want the school to have something to build on. If a child can't recognize letters and numbers and does not have beginning reading skills, school districts will often place them in severe-needs classrooms where academics come second to behavior and diagnosis. There are instances when the school can teach a nonverbal or semi-verbal child to read and write, but in my experience, I've found that when children can't read they get pushed through special education classes that focus on behavior and not learning.

Some kids with autism pick up reading and writing on their own or at school; in which case you will not have to teach core academics. For those kids maybe behavior or speech therapy is a more appropriate intervention. Regardless of where your child is academically, it is important to support the school by addressing deficits and/or behaviors, so your child can be successful in an academic setting.

In some cases, a child with autism will not qualify for an IEP but will qualify for a 504 plan. A 504 plan provides protections under IDEA. Children who are minimally affected by autism may fall under the umbrella of the ADA via a 504 plan. This plan ensures a *free* *appropriate* *public* *education* (FAPE) under the ADA and will provide minimal accommodations for students with autism or other disabilities. A 504 plan does not require multiple lengthy meetings like an IEP meeting does, and written documentation is not always a requirement with a 504 plan (although some school district choose to put the plans in writing).

Our job as parents isn't to educate our kids from kindergarten through twelfth grade (unless you homeschool). Instead, our job is to help prepare our kids for academic success. We can help prepare them by teaching them the basics of math and reading. We can also help prepare them for the classroom by hiring behavior therapists, OTs, or SLPs. Regardless of where our kids fall on the spectrum, there are always opportunities for us to support them and prepare them for academic success. We don't have to be college professors or scholars to help our kids get ready for the classroom; we just have to be creative, pay attention to their particular learning style, and come up with ways to help them succeed academically.

PREPARE FOR THE IEP

IEP meetings aren't always fun. I have had IEP meetings where everything went well, the teachers, and support staff had excellent ideas, and I felt comfortable with their recommendations. On the other hand, I have had IEP meetings where we yelled at each other and didn't agree on placement, David's level of functioning, or his learning capabilities. Basically, we didn't agree on anything.

David has been in seven schools. One preschool, three elementary schools, two middle schools, and he just started high school this year. Preschool was great, but the first two elementary schools were a nightmare, and the third school was phenomenal. His first year of middle school was a joke. His teacher hadn't read his IEP and had him learning the alphabet when he was capable of reading (close to) grade-level text. They closed that school and put him in a different middle school where the teachers were invested in his education and worked to get him caught up. High school has been interesting. His school is genuinely trying to support his needs as well as accommodate his tenacious and feisty mother. Every school is different and, because we never know what we're walking into, it's critically important we are well prepared for IEP meetings. A solid IEP can mean the difference between a quality education and glorified babysitting.

An IEP is geared toward the child as an individual. One child with autism may need OT, SLP, PT, and a one-on-one aide, while another child with autism may only need help with organizing their planner and social skills. Each child is different and has different needs. The IEP is meant to support the child based on their individual needs and not the blanket diagnosis of autism.

When preparing for the IEP, there is basic information you will want to know ahead of time. Acronyms will most likely be used, so you can photocopy the list of acronyms provided or take this book with you. You should also know your state's law with regard to voice recordings.[8] In Colorado, I can record all IEP meetings because we are a "one-party consent" state, meaning only one party has to know he or she is being recorded. The purpose of recording is to ensure that your school district sticks to the promises they make during the IEP.

When I had my first IEP meeting for David, I could not have imagined recording meetings. Now I can't imagine not recording a meeting, and with today's smartphones recording a meeting is simple. I have been promised the sun, moon, and stars during IEP meetings just to be given a lump of coal. Let me give you an example of what I mean. David's first elementary school would eventually go from bad to worse the year after the kids were moved back into the building. The following year David was in first grade. School seemed to be going okay at first; he had a new teacher, and some of the aides were new.

After a couple months into the school year, he'd start to cry when I'd put him on the bus for school in the morning. I didn't think much of it because unexplained behaviors were just a part of our lives. I initially thought it was a sensory response I witnessed some things at his school that were disturbing. I started reading about special education law and found a federal statute that said I can go into his school at any time, unannounced. So I did. I started going to school with him every day.

I went to school with him for over two years. The school he was in was not educating him. David did very little academics during the school day and at the time I thought this was normal. I thought the system marginalized our kids and there wasn't much a parent could do to change things. Every attempt I made to increase learning time was met with resistance.

I was done begging them to educate him. I was done with getting the cold shoulder from the aides and teachers. I was done fighting for an education he wasn't getting. I called the district to put in a request to transfer schools.

We had a meeting and put David in another school. I knew it was not the right placement for him, but I tried to make it work. Then one day I got a call from the school asking why David was not there. I said, "I put him on the bus myself this morning. He'd better be there. Check the classrooms again. I'll call the police." My ex-husband and I ran to the car and sped to his school. On the way there I called the Transportation Department and told them to check his bus and make sure he wasn't on it. The Transportation Department called me back a few minutes later and said he was on the bus. That was about 10:00 a.m. I had put him on the bus at 7:50, which means he was on a parked school bus in the cold, in December, for over two hours.

When the bus pulled up, there were police waiting there, and they were the first to see him. The police officer looked at me and said, "He doesn't look good." As David came around the back of the police officer, his little face and hands were covered in blood and he looked terrified. He had gotten so nervous he scratched his face until it bled. The bus driver said when he found David he was sitting on the steps of the bus scratching his face. It was quite a scene. My husband (at the time) looked like he was about to pass out, David was a bloody mess, the police needed a report from me, the school staff were freaking out, and I had to hold it together.

When I went into the school to talk to the police and staff, the Director of Transportation called and asked me what I wanted to do about the bus driver. I responded, "Well, at the end of the day, my family and I live in a bubble. People stare at us in the store, doctors don't like me to bring my son into their office, we don't get invited to anything, and your driver is one of the only people who is nice to my son. She buys him little treats he can have and gave him a Christmas present. She is one of the only people who is happy to see him and who is kind to us. If you are asking me if I want her fired, the answer is no. She should be disciplined, but I do not want her fired. I assume she learned a lesson and this won't happen again." Was I upset with the driver? Of course, but in truth, she loved David and would never intend to hurt him. She later called me crying hysterically and said, "I may lose my job, and I don't care if I do. I am so worried about David. Is he okay? Can I do anything to help? Please tell him I'm sorry. I love that kid." While I was upset about the incident, I used it as an opportunity to increase awareness in the district.

I insisted that all bus drivers and bus aides in our area (I live in a huge county that is divided up into articulation areas) receive autism education and training. This one incident created an opportunity to increase awareness and make sure all drivers and aides were aware of how vulnerable our kids really are. Needless to say, he did not stay at that school. I put in another request to transfer and scheduled a transition meeting to talk about which schools were available. At the transition meeting, there were lawyers, the head of special education for my area, several special education employees from the district, two teachers, school therapists, a general education teacher, myself, my advocate, and Cindy (David's OT at the time).

The transition meeting occurred shortly after the bus incident, and I was still a hot mess. In truth, David being left on the bus was emotionally crippling for me. I was so scared of him going to school I couldn't sleep well at night and felt drained all day. I was scared of him being lost again, and I could barely function for about a month after he was left on the bus. I stayed in bed all day and got up two hours before the kids came home to take a shower and clean the house to try and keep up appearances. It devastated me, my ex, and our relationship. We were both changed by that experience as I'm sure David was, but at the time he couldn't speak very much and couldn't tell us how he felt. We both constantly reassured him he would be safe and that his new bus driver would be more careful (although secretly we were both apprehensive about his safety).

Back to the transition meeting, I had asked an educational advocate to come with me to the meeting as I knew I was too fragile to articulate a solid argument for his placement. When we got to the meeting, Cindy and I sat at one end of the table, and my advocate sat at the other end of the table with the head of special education for my area. I thought it was unusual for my advocate to sit at the other end of the table because we couldn't talk about anything if she wasn't sitting next to me, but nevertheless, I tried to stay positive, focused on David's placement. We agreed on a transfer to a really great school on the other end of town. The issue with that particular school was that it did not have a fence. Because David wandered at the time (and had been forgotten about and left on a bus), I was scared to send him to that particular school because it did not have a fence and was on a large lot in close proximity to busy streets.

Here is where I learned a valuable lesson about IEP and transition meetings. I was not recording the meeting and when I asked the district head to put up a fence she said she'd have to look at the budget and decide from there. I looked at my advocate (who was sitting next to the district head) and said, "He can't go there without a fence. Wandering is the leading cause of death for people with autism. Aren't you going to say something?" My advocate said, "It should be fine. They have supervision outside." To which I responded, "They have two aides getting them off the bus and a bus driver who said she checked the bus after she dropped off the kids and he wasn't on there. Things happen; supervision does not guarantee his safety. I need a fence up to protect him and the other kids with autism." She literally was not listening as she and the district head were looking at a cell phone, laughing at something.

I started crying and kept saying, "He could die. What are you thinking?" My advocate did and said nothing, and finally David's OT said, "We need to call this meeting. Obviously, we can't reach an agreement and should address this another time." We left, and after I pulled myself together I scheduled a meeting for the next week with the head of special education for my area and another special education supervisor. At that meeting the district head agreed to put up a fence but refused to put it in writing. I didn't record the meeting, and with nothing in writing, lo and behold, she would not return my calls and clearly had no intention of putting up a fence. I went to the school principal and asked her to put up a fence. She said the school had the funds and she would have it built but needed the district to sign off on it.

Guess what? The district would not sign off on construction and would not return my calls or emails. What did I do? I went to the news again, and they came out and did a story on the school. I had bake sales and garage sales and the news story reported that I had received enough donations to have a fence put up at David's school, and the district finally agreed to allow construction at the school.

What I learned from these experiences is that it is important to record meetings. Without a recording school districts can make promises and not keep them. Each state has different laws pertaining to recording meetings, so as I said you should clarify your state laws before recording an IEP meeting. I also learned that not all advocates are good advocates. After that experience I set out to learn special education law on my own to avoid ever needing an advocate again.

I also learned that it's important to set the tone of an IEP meeting before it starts. I no longer bring David to IEP meetings if I feel we need to discuss his deficits. It is not healthy for our children to sit through two hours of hearing about everything they do wrong. I also start each IEP meeting by stating that I would like to keep the tone of the meeting positive and focus on ways to build on David's strengths and not focus on his weaknesses.

I learned a lot form the bus incident. I learned that people do not always follow through on their duties (bus drivers in my county are required to check the bus for kids before they exit the bus and sign off; she signed off as having checked the bus, but clearly she didn't), and I learned that there are many people who work in special education who have no experience educating children with autism. I learned that I had to be my son's advocate even though it meant spending an entire summer poring over law books.

In preparing for the IEP, it is important to know your child's rights under IDEA. I also encourage parents to read the book *How to Win Friends and Influence People*[9] before attending a contentious IEP meeting. This particular book explains how to negotiate effectively while building strong relationships with the people with whom you interact. It's helpful to be well organized and write down your main points and relevant statutes before entering an IEP meeting. These meetings can get emotional, so it is important to have your ideas written down to keep you on track.

I also believe it is important to go to IEP meetings dressed professionally. Although I don't think it's fair to judge a person based on how they dress, the reality is that people do judge us based on our appearances. It's important to be presentable for IEP or transition meetings. I am not saying you need to wear a ball gown or tuxedo. What I am saying is that people will take you more seriously if you come to the meeting looking presentable.

LEARN HOW TO RESOLVE EDUCATIONAL CONFLICT

Conflict resolution as it pertains to special education can be tricky business. Avoiding conflict by being professional, kind, and polite is always best. If that does not get you very far, you will need to know how to fight and how to win. In terms of conflict resolution, there are several avenues you can take to address the issue at hand. If you think your child would benefit from social skills classes and more support in the classroom, for example, and the district declines your request, you can have your child's therapists and/or pediatrician write a letter stating the benefits of such support. If that doesn't work, request an **emergency IEP** meeting. An emergency IEP meeting must be held within twenty-four school hours after the request was made. Always email your request so you have a written record. If the issues are not resolved in the emergency IEP meeting, file a complaint.

Each school district has unique methods of addressing complaints, so call the special education department in your school district and ask how to file a complaint. If that doesn't work, file a complaint with the Department of Education in your state. When you write your complaint, try to suspend emotion and stick to the facts. For example, "My son's pediatrician and therapist have recommended additional support in the classroom to ensure my child can access the curriculum. The additional support will enable him to complete assignments and stay on track academically. I believe this to be a reasonable accommodation as defined in the Americans with Disabilities Act." You will want to stick to the law and present the case that this support or intervention will allow your child to access grade-level curricula and ensure adherence to FAPE.

If a situation at school is not being resolved and the district is not in compliance with the law, you can request **mediation**. I personally have not gone this route for myself because mediation can be binding, and I didn't want to be in a situation where I didn't have a say in his education. However, mediation has served other families well, and the mediator is, or should be, an independent third party. A good mediator will help parents and the school district come to a consensus.

If a situation arises and suspension, expulsion, or disciplinary actions are taken by the school district, you will need to establish a *behavior intervention plan* (BIP). A BIP is basically an addition to the IEP which outlines effective behavioral interventions and strategies. The BIP includes parent reports and recommendations from the child's therapists and pediatricians if applicable. The BIP will often call for an FBA to determine which interventions are most effective. Most of our kids would benefit from a BIP, and if your child does not have one, you can request that the child's teacher or case manager start the process.

In cases where disciplinary actions are being considered (suspension over ten days, expulsion, etc.), a **manifestation determination** is required for children with an IEP. A manifestation determination is basically the school district and parents sitting down together to determine if the child's behavior is a manifestation of the child's disability or not. In most cases, kids who have autism misbehave as a direct result of their disability; they are not being malicious or intentionally misbehaving. As our kids get older, manifestation determinations are needed for a different purpose. Unfortunately, there are times when our kids are talked into doing bad things by typical peers. When this happens, our kids are often punished without the implementation of a manifestation determination. If your child ends up in hot water at school, especially if the police are involved, request a manifestation determination.

Once you have requested this, the teacher and possibly district personnel will most likely want to meet with you. When you have a meeting about behavior, it's important to bring statements or doctors' notes on your child's emotional and developmental state. Your job in this instance is to demonstrate that your child's behavior is a manifestation of their disability. Letters from therapists or scholarly journals supporting your case should be taken into consideration during this process. It is possible you will be met with resistance because school district personnel typically have very little training in autism. My school district tells me no and disagrees with me frequently. I pay it no mind. My advice is to do your research, get organized, and dig your heels in; don't back down. Our kids are so innocent; the idea of them being punished for behavior is in most cases absurd and grossly irresponsible on the part of the school district.

In your quest to make sure your child receives a quality education, there will be a need for evaluations and reevaluations. I have had parents tell me they don't want to consent to the evaluations. In that case they have the right to seek an independent evaluation and hope the district recognizes it. It is important to clarify which professionals your district recognizes as experts for the particular issue you are facing. For me, I have always agreed to allow our school district to conduct evaluations because I have met the people who do them and trust their judgment. However you decide to go about evaluations is your choice, just know that evaluations are a part of establishing a solid IEP or sometimes a 504 plan.

There are minor issues with school districts, and then there are major, Goliath-sized issues. For minor matters, emergency IEP meetings, adding a BIP or going through evaluations can address most issues that come up. If you have tried everything and it hasn't worked, if you have been kind, gracious, and understanding and that didn't work, if you have done everything in your power to work with the school and it didn't work, it's time for the major league. If you enter the major league of conflict resolution with your school district, you will need to be brave and you will need to be bold. I know that we sometimes feel tired, defeated and unable to keep fighting, but as Winston Churchill said, "If you're going through hell, just keep going." Just keep going.

There are times when you will need to go big. If you have exhausted all avenues and your child is being bullied, denied FAPE or discriminated against, you may need to file an OCR. An OCR is short for an Office for Civil Rights complaint. This type of complaint is reserved for civil rights violations only. For example, when David's class was moved to the temporary buildings and segregated from the general population, I could have filed a civil rights complaint for discrimination based on his disability, but I was not aware of OCR complaints at the time. If, for example, your child is punished at school and was suspended for more than ten days, or charges were pressed by the school and the school failed to do a manifestation determination and implement a BIP, you may have a case for an OCR violation. If you believe your child's civil rights (the Americans with Disabilities Act prohibits discrimination against people with disabilities in public places) were violated, you will want to pursue this type of complaint. To file an OCR violation, you will want to go online and fill out the applicable forms.[10] If you do not have access to a computer or internet, you can call 800-421-3481 and tell them you would like to file an OCR/Department of Education complaint and ask for the address to mail in the complaint in your state. You have 180 days to file your complaint, although the sooner you file, the better. School districts that discriminate against our kids do so habitually. They will not self-correct. It often takes parents with gumption to get them to change their policies. That parent might be you.

If you believe your child, or any person with a disability for that matter, has been discriminated against, you can submit a complaint and the OCR will evaluate the complaint and determine if they have grounds to investigate. If they believe they have the authority to investigate, they will contact you and you can move your case forward.

Filing an OCR complaint is a big deal. If an institution, person, or business has violated a person's civil rights and the OCR finds they are in noncompliance with federal law, they can lose federal funding, they can be fined, and they may have to make significant changes to their programs. Filing an OCR is not something you would do on a whim. It is reserved only for cases of clear discrimination. In my mind, the purpose of filing an OCR on behalf of a person with autism is to get school districts to change policies and procedures when it comes to educating kids with autism.

I feel that fines and loss of federal funding would hurt our kids as funding for education is insufficient as it stands. The goal of this complaint is to get your school district in compliance with federal laws pertaining to IDEA and the ADA so that your child, and the kids who come after him or her, can receive a quality public education.

If you have exhausted all options and your child is still not being educated properly, you can file due process. Even I, after everything that has happened with David at school, have not filed due process. Due process is, well, a nightmare for parents. It can drag on for years, it can cost thousands of dollars in lawyers' fees, and it does not always work in favor of the child (if you lose your case). Although filing due process is still on the table for us, I have avoided it like the plague as I don't have the money to hire an attorney. Many parents are in my shoes; they want to file and ask their school district to pay for private school but can't afford an attorney.

In my case, I know the law well enough to represent David myself, but even then it would be tough for me as I'd be learning the system from the ground up (something I should be used to by now). Despite the fact that I know the law and I'm fastidious and well-spoken, I would be up against the district's high-powered, experienced team of attorneys. The odds are not in my favor. It is difficult for parents to win these cases. Although due process is not fun or easy, it is necessary in certain circumstances.

Before you file a due process complaint, you will want to make sure you have attempted to resolve the issue(s) in an IEP meeting. You may also want to consider mediation before filing due process if you think it's appropriate.

Parents file due process for a number of reasons, but in many cases, we are filing due process after years of attempting to get our school districts to comply with federal statutes under IDEA. In my case if I were to file due process, it would be because I do not feel my school district is capable of providing my son with an appropriate education. If I were to file due process, it would be contingent upon a violation of IDEA and my complaint would need to be filed within two years of the violation.

If a parent hires an attorney and wins the case, in many instances attorney's fees incurred during the process can be granted. If you choose to represent your child yourself or cannot afford an attorney, you can file a due process complaint notice on your own. The complaint notice, which can be filed by a parent *or* school district, clearly outlines the specific violations and provides reasonable solutions to resolve the issue at hand.

When filing due process parents will need to give the school a copy of the complaint. The burden of proof falls on the party making the complaint. You will need to compile school documents, pertinent emails and correspondence, and letters from physicians and therapists if needed, and ultimately, prove your child's rights were violated under IDEA.

It is a complex process. If you feel due process is necessary, you will want to speak to an attorney or advocate who works specifically with special education law. Although parents can file due process on their own, it is important to know your rights and run your complaint notice by an attorney or advocate before filing.

Ensuring that children with autism receive a quality education comes down to two factors: one, parents helping to establish core academic skills like reading and number recognition (if necessary), and two, parents knowing the basics of special education law. Like everything else pertaining to autism, parents need to be vigilant and focused on the goal. If your child is to receive a quality education, you are a vital piece of that puzzle. Stay vigilant and never give up!

NOTES FOR CHAPTER 6

7

PREPARING YOUR CHILD FOR ADOLESCENCE AND ADULTHOOD

But I ask you, those of you who are with us all day, not to stress yourselves out because of us. When you do this, it feels as if you're denying any value at all that our lives may have—and that saps the spirit we need to soldier on. The hardest ordeal for us is the idea that we are causing grief for other people. We can put up with our own hardships okay, but the thought that our lives are the source of other people's unhappiness, that's plain unbearable.

—Naoki Higashida[1]

WHEN NAOKI HIGASHIDA wrote the book *The Reason I Jump*, he was thirteen years old. As our children grow into adolescents, they need more encouragement, praise, and support than ever before. It is at this critical stage in their development that we need to build them into strong adults. They may seem aloof, but children with autism are generally aware of and absorb everything around them. As they enter adulthood the words that are said to them either build up or tear down the foundation of their self-esteem. It is at this time in their lives, the awkward teenage years, that they need the most structure and love. As they grow, their awareness of the world around them grows as well.

The teenage years are even tougher for kids with autism than they are for typical kids. There will be hormones, a roller coaster of emotions, and in our case a whole lot of dirty looks and eye rolls. Having a young child with autism presents one set of challenges; having a teenage child with autism comes with an entirely different set of challenges. As our kids grow they need to be taught activities of daily living, life skills, money management, hygiene, and everything in between.

As they grow into adults, our expectations of our kids should grow accordingly. The world around them expects them to have manners, proper social etiquette, good hygiene, and the ability to communicate on some level. Some of our kids will be able to live independently, and some won't. Our role, as arduous as it may seem, is to prepare them for as much independence as possible depending upon where they fall on the spectrum.

Like in the poem I quoted at the top of chapter 5, a child's greatest need is to be needed, and this is especially true of children with autism. Accomplishing day-to-day activities can help build their self-esteem and establish feelings of self-worth.

All of our kids have potential. They have the potential to communicate, the potential to learn new skills, and the potential to completely and wildly exceed our expectations. For this chapter we will focus on building on our children's strengths and learn ways to help prepare them for adolescence and adulthood. Here's what we'll be covering:

- Build communication skills
- Teach essential life skills
- Work on safety skills
- Teach basic home repairs
- Prepare your child for puberty

BUILD COMMUNICATION SKILLS

As our kids grow into teenagers and eventually adults, there are certain skills they must have in order to function at their highest level. Communication is one of those skills. Because the autism spectrum is so broad, the best way to teach communication skills is to build on the child's existing vocabulary. Some children with autism never speak, but there are children with autism who cannot speak who are capable of writing blogs and entire books, like Carly (the young lady I referenced in chapter 3). No matter where your child lands on the spectrum, there is always the possibility they can communicate.

Determining the best mode of communication depends on where your child is on the spectrum and what his or her communication needs are. If your child is nonverbal, I suggest teaching them the song I mentioned in chapter 6. The song is an excellent way to introduce word cards and facilitate communication. Once they have built upon word recognition, they can use word cards to communicate their needs or transfer this skill to a computer or tablet. If you believe picture cards and the PECS system is best, build on picture-based communication skills. Even when a child is nonverbal it does not mean they are incapable of communicating; they just need creative means to do so.[2]

For children who are semi-verbal (like David), parents can hire a speech therapist and/or add communication skills to the goals for behavior therapy. With the right support from therapists, our kids can learn how to communicate essential needs and begin to establish conversational skills. David is just now starting to say things like, "How was your day, Mother?" or "Hello, Mom and brothers, how was sledding?" David's vocabulary expands a little more each week, and with the help of his dedicated therapists, his communication skills are improving significantly.

David learned to read and write before he could talk, and his language base was enormous by the time he began to speak in sentences. Our kids are in there, absorbing everything that is said around them. With the right support they can learn to communicate in their own way.

If a child is high functioning, communication comes with an entirely unique set of challenges. High-functioning kids with autism need to learn how to interact and socialize, and part of that is learning how to have back-and-forth conversations. High-functioning kids need support as they enter adolescence because they will want to make friends at school and will, in most cases, need adequate guidance in order to do so.

Let's say, for example, your child has high-functioning autism and is obsessed with trains. Each person met will hear about their love of trains, and while I think that's adorable, that may not be well-received in middle school. Focusing on functional communication with a qualified therapist can help our kids learn how to engage in meaningful back-and-forth conversations. If you so choose you can add functional communication to your child's IEP goals. Many schools offer social skills groups to help with peer interactions and build vocabulary.

If you are struggling to find ways to help your child communicate, TACA has excellent resources for kids on the spectrum. They list everything from apps for autism to PECS and offer really great advice on increasing communication.[3]

As an example of how important communication can be as children grow up, last school year David was sent home three times in a month because he vomited. He vomited a couple times at home, but because he has severe allergies, I thought he was sneaking food. He then started complaining of headaches, so I took him to his doctor's office and explained that he'd been saying, "My head hurts, ouch, ouch, ouch," every day for a week. The pediatrician said migraines often start in puberty and can cause vomiting in some cases. He recommended I put David on magnesium and increase his water intake. After a few weeks of him taking magnesium and drinking tons of water, his headaches disappeared, and the vomiting went with it.

Now imagine if David were nonverbal and had no way to communicate. Doctors would go through a number of tests, probably do blood work (we ended up doing three blood draws to rule out other conditions), maybe an MRI and possibly add medication to stop the vomiting. David's ability to communicate, although minimal, enabled me and his doctor to pinpoint the root cause of his symptoms, and the issue was resolved quickly.

Although communication can be difficult to teach, it is of the utmost importance that our kids have *some* ability to express themselves, even if it is simply signing a few words. David learned basic sign language when he was nonverbal, and it allowed him to ask for a drink, tell me when he needed to eat, and say "hello," "goodbye," "I love you," "more," "thank you," and "help." Even learning a minimal amount of sign language can allow children to express themselves and communicate their needs. Reaching out to the experts and thinking outside the box (like using RPM, for instance, as mentioned in chapter 5) can help you bridge this gap. There is always a way to increase vocabulary, and it is at this critical stage in their lives that communication is most needed. Never give up!

TEACH ESSENTIAL LIFE SKILLS

TACA has an incredible "Essential Life Skills Chart" which is available online and cited in the endnotes, is very helpful for parents as our children mature. My best advice is to print out the chart and keep it on the fridge or somewhere you will see it on a daily basis. Sometimes, a simple visual reminder of what our goals are can keep us on track.

As your child enters middle and high school, he or she will most likely start to work on independent living skills at school. If you feel this chart is helpful, you can add sections of it to your child's IEP.[4]

I realize that many of us grow accustomed to doing just about everything for our kids. It can be hard to imagine they can do household chores and complete activities of daily living (ADLs) on their own. I did literally everything for David until I read "Beatitudes for Friends of Disabled Children." I realized then that David wants to be a part of things and contribute to the household. Once I started asking him to help me, I saw a change in his demeanor. He started to smile more and seemed to be empowered by helping his mom; it gave him the self-esteem he needed to try new tasks around the house.

At this point David does just as many chores as his brother, Aidan. He unloads the dishwasher, he does his own laundry, and he is learning to dust and vacuum. He is now very organized and puts his DVDs and video games back on the shelf every time (they used to be scattered all over the house). It took patience and lots of time to teach him these skills, but eventually he got the hang of them and he is now conscientious about cleaning up after himself.

I also think that perspective is vitally important when we begin to teach our children new life skills. If we go into it knowing that teaching these skills will require patience and time, the process will go a bit more smoothly. A parent's perspective and attitude oftentimes determine how much progress a child will make in this area. If we are encouraging, positive, and supportive, our kids stand a much better chance of gaining new skills. If we are negative and critical during this process, it will hinder their ability to make gains.

It took months to teach David how to do his own laundry and unload the dishwasher, but now that he's got it down, he helps me with the dishes just about every day. He is learning new skills around the house, and yes, it's taking time, but he'll get that soon enough too. My goal is not to bombard him with expectations but instead, teach him a new skill every few months. When he moves into his own place someday, I want him to know how to care for himself and keep his home in order.

Teaching a child with autism to pick up after themselves and to do chores requires patience (like Mother-Teresa-type patience) and may require advice from an OT or behavior therapist. However you go about teaching these skills is up to you, but if your child is capable of doing any chores at all, it will benefit them in the long run to do so. When they grow up and age into adult services, they will be expected to help clean their own home, do laundry, grocery shop, etc. If a child with autism is not taught these life skills, they will most likely be in their service plan as an adult. By then, these tasks can seem overwhelming.

The chart from TACA also lists **financial literacy** as an essential life skill. If your child has a special needs trust fund and is in any way capable of monitoring his own finances, he will need to learn how manage money, how to self-advocate, and know who to contact if there are issues with the trust. If your child grows up and does not have a trust and is dependent upon government assistance, he will need to know how to budget, as food stamps are very minimal for adults with disabilities. They will have limited funds through Social Security and will need to know how to budget money effectively before entering into adult services.

Financial literacy can be hard to teach our kids. You can include this in your child's IEP as a goal for math. You will want to word it in a way that is consistent with IEP goals, such as, "David will learn to balance a checkbook accurately with minimal assistance 75% of the time (something like that)." You can also reach out to your OT and/or BCBA and ask to add financial literacy to your child's therapy goals.

I struggle teaching financial literacy to David. Money is an abstract concept for him to grasp, and he simply isn't ready to take this on quite yet. Despite the fact that he is not ready to manage money, I continue to take steps to enhance his money-management skills. One way I approach this is to have him sit down with me while I write out my budget for the month. This way he sees what our monthly bills are and how much money from each paycheck goes toward bills and what is left over for recreational activities.

I try to teach financial literacy by including David in our everyday financial decisions. For example, when we go grocery shopping I tell him, "We have $250 for groceries this week, and this food has to last us until next week; think about what you'll need for school lunches, snacks, and meals." I can see the wheels turning in his brilliant mind as he grabs a cart and goes and shops for himself. He isn't ready to manage the grocery money quite yet, but I am taking steps to get him used to meal planning and budgeting.

Health and wellness are included in the chart, and I believe these are among the most important skills we can teach our kids. As they turn into teenagers, kids need to learn proper hygiene and grooming. This particular skill set is necessary for health reasons but social reasons as well. Kids can be mean, and if a child with autism is picked on for having stinky armpits or for wearing dirty clothes to school, that hurt can stick with them for a lifetime. Personal appearance is important if they want to maintain employment, have roommates, date etc. Appearance is more than materialism; it is about teaching them to care for and respect their body.

Health and wellness includes basic first aid, maintaining a healthy diet, safety and exercise. These skills, in most cases, will not come naturally to kids with autism. As they mature their therapy and IEP goals should start to include essential life skills. Some of these skills can be taught at school but may easily be taught at home. One example is diet. Children often mirror the eating habits of their primary caregiver. Although many kids with autism have

sensory issues around food, a good OT or speech therapist can help decrease oral sensory sensitivity and can open
them up to trying new foods. Once the sensory piece has
been addressed, parents can start to add in healthier food
choices during meals and snacks. In time these choices will
become a habit they can carry into adulthood. Establishing
good eating habits doesn't have to be grueling. You can do
small things like eating organic fruit leathers instead of the
processed versions people commonly buy. I make the kids
organic fruit smoothies and while David only drinks a tiny
bit, he is starting to enjoy them. It's a clever way to incorporate fruits and/or vegetables into the diet.

Prescription drugs are a part of health and wellness
education. If a child takes medication every day, he will
need to know how to monitor the meds, order them, and
budget for the cost if living independently. If these skills
are taught, there is the potential for some of our kids to
manage their own medications when we are no longer able
to care for them.

I'll admit the Essential Life Skills chart is a bit intimidating, but this is not something you have to tackle alone; you
can always bring the chart to your child's next IEP meeting
if your child is twelve or older and ask which of these skills
can be worked on at school. I know that in my school district, cooking, laundry, dishes and public transportation can
all be taught during the school day if included in the IEP.

Teaching essential life skills is made easier by adding
one thing at a time and breaking each skill down into small,
attainable goals. If you want to teach how to use the naviga-
tion app on your phone, show your little angel how it works
and let him hold it while you drive. If you want to teach the
importance of landmarks, it's as simple as pointing things
out while you drive. Remember, I taught David the alphabet
and how to read at a time when he almost never looked
at me; just because they aren't looking at us, doesn't necessarily mean they aren't paying attention. Teaching new

skills can be as simple as keeping our kids close by while we go through our everyday routines. Teaching life skills does not have to be an arduous task. We can incorporate these lessons in our everyday lives.

There are a few things on the list that are a bit overwhelming for me as a mom, like **transportation** for example. I can't imagine teaching David to drive, but I know that someday he will be able to do so, and I will need to teach him everything that comes with the responsibility of owning and operating a vehicle. Although he isn't ready to drive, I can teach him how to put gas in the car, how to fill the windshield washer fluid reservoir and how to check fluids and air pressure in the tires. My best advice is to simply do a little at a time and have fun doing it. Your child will love spending the time with you and will appreciate your belief in his ability to learn new things.

I realize that not all people with autism have the ability to drive. Some of our kids will benefit from learning bus routes and how to navigate public transportation. In many secondary autism programs, kids have the opportunity to take the bus with their teachers and classmates for practice. Transportation can also be a behavior therapy goal; however, some agencies don't allow therapists to take clients in public. If your therapist is on board and their agency supports it, they can help your child learn bus routes to and from any given location. If not, this is another opportunity for parents and children to bond while learning a new essential life skill.

Another essential life skill that needs to be addressed is **employment**. As our children become adolescents, it's important to hone in on their interests and skill set. David, for example, loves animals and is fascinated by computers. When we go to the park, my other two boys run, jump, swing and play while David often sits on the ground, away from the noise of the playground, and waits for the geese to come to him (my city has hundreds of lakes, and geese are a part of almost every park experience for us). Animals love him, and he is at peace around them. Working with animals would be very therapeutic for David.

On the other hand, he has the ability to navigate computers better than the average person. When he was six, my Dad's computer had the dreaded blue screen of death and was inoperable. David went downstairs to my Dad's office, and after some time I went down to check on him. He had my Dad's computer up and running and was watching YouTube videos. David is exceptionally skilled at fixing computer issues and can remember URLs that are fifty characters long.

As I start to plan for his future, he and I have conversations about where he wants to work and what he wants to do. So far, it's a tie between working at the zoo to, in his words, "hug the animals" and designing video games. Because coding and video game production can be lucrative, I am hoping he'll lean toward that career path. A local university offers coding classes for teenagers with autism in the summer, and I'm hoping he'll agree to go. Building skills for employment is something we can do gradually. In time, their interests will come to light, and we can start to prepare our kids for a career they are passionate about. No matter what your child is interested in, there is always a market for dedicated employees.

Sometimes it's difficult to establish what work would be suitable for our children and what they would enjoy doing. If you are struggling to pinpoint which type of work your child would enjoy, there is an online tool called the Marquette Strengths Index that can help guide you.[5] The Marquette Strengths Index is used to help people with autism and other disabilities establish which career choices will suit them best. The Index asks a series of questions, and from the answers, the client is given a number of career choices that complement their skills.

Also keep in mind that your local disability resource center should have vocational training classes available for your child; age requirements vary state to state, but most adult service programs start at age eighteen. These classes will help your child build on existing skills and learn proper etiquette when applying for jobs. These classes can also help young adults who have autism learn social skills, how to fill out an application, and how to write a resume. Additionally, some school districts partner with trade schools. If your district partners with local trade schools, your child may have the opportunity to participate in trade programs while in high school. The trade school near us offers computer courses, welding, construction, coding and auto mechanics. There are a number of courses David can take to prepare him for adulthood and help him learn skills that will make him more self-sufficient.

As our children become adults, they will need to be taught everything we do in our day-to-day lives, including **social and recreational** activities. As the mother of a teenage boy with autism, this has been one of the hardest issues I've had to tackle. He wants to get out and socialize, make friends, go to the mall (minus his mom), go to parties, hang out with girls, and maintain relationships with kids his age. I struggle with this for a number of reasons. I am wary of new people around him because of all of the bad things that happened to him in the past while in the care of others. My fears, although well founded, make it very difficult for me to allow him freedoms.

The desire to socialize is heightened in middle and high school. David has been in several schools, and it's been difficult for him to make friends because he is never in one school for long. Lately, he's been tearing up and saying, "I fail at people. Where are my friends?" If he were not able to communicate, those emotions would surely come across in the form of negative behaviors. Although his communication is still limited, he can tell me how he feels and what he's thinking, which has helped to eliminate negative behaviors. Although he doesn't pal around with kids at school, the truth is that he does have friends, and now that I know it bothers him, I have made a point to get him together with his buddies when we have free time.

Since David has expressed a need to socialize with other kids, I have consulted his BCBA. David's BCBA is brilliant, and he's made some excellent recommendations to help David through this. We're going to start a calendar for David, so when he starts to perseverate over hanging out with friends, I can reference the calendar and he'll know that, for example, in two weeks we'll go to the movies with a friend, and the week after that we'll go to the mall with a different friend. Using a calendar as a visual reminder will help him in two ways: one, he can see the dates he'll be meeting up with other kids and feel at ease about his social life; and two, it gives him something positive to think about. Using a calendar will give him a visual reminder of the fact that he does have friends, and it gives him something to look forward to. David's BCBA also suggested I take pictures of our outings with friends and print them out for David. When he starts to get upset, we can reference the pictures and it will give him a sense of peace knowing that he does have other teenagers to hang out with.

Making friends is challenging for adolescents on the spectrum, and sometimes parents have to take some initiative to make those relationships possible. Last year I reached out to David's teacher and asked if she could pass my email address on to other parents who were interested in getting their children together for social activities. David made a good friend from my doing this. They both love Jump Street, an indoor trampoline park, and movies. It's a perfect match! When David had his fifteenth birthday party, I invited every kid in his class, and lo and behold, enough kids showed up to make it a party. I made sure to get the parents' phone numbers in order for us to get together, and it worked! David hangs out with the kids from the party from time to time as well. On top of that a neurotypical child from David's elementary school goes places with us on occasion and David loves every minute of it. The last time we dropped his NT friend off at home after a night out, David said with tears in his eyes, "Thanks for the school reunion, Mom."

Sometimes, in order for our kids to socialize, we need to directly influence the process. Many parents are struggling to match their kids up with peers, and it can be as easy as reaching out to your child's teacher or therapists and asking if they know of other parents who are interested in getting the kids together. I recently discovered an app called Meetup I intend to try. This app allows people with autism to find social activities or pair up with a buddy. As parents, we always have the option of creating a Facebook group for teenagers with autism; once we've established the group, we can reach out to our local Autism Society, Parent to Parent, and our child's teachers and therapists to find members to join. No matter what the issue is, with a little creative thinking and ingenuity, we can help our kids acquire essential life skills, including social skills.

There is also a clear and purposeful need to teach our children manners as they grow into adulthood. We get so used to our kid's behavior and quirks that we often overlook little things they do. Unfortunately, their behavior can be perceived by others as bad manners. Teaching good manners has no downside and will allow for more social opportunities. If we want our kids to make friends, have sleepovers, and be able to hang out at a buddy's house, we must instill the importance of social graces.

I don't think children with autism need to have perfect manners, but they should be able to go to a person's house and show respect for their things and for their privacy. For example, if your child has a habit of opening the bathroom door when you're in there, that may not be a big deal at home, but it could have long-term negative effects on their ability to form new friendships. If a child opens up the cupboards and refrigerator and helps himself to food at home, that's great, but it may not be well received at a friend's house.

Teaching manners is a crucial step in a child's development. Good manners and social graces can get a person farther than just about anything else. Teaching social graces and good manners will make life a bit easier for our kids. David learned to say please and thank you as soon as he could speak. He shares, he cleans up after himself, and he is, in general, very respectful of other's personal space and property. Because David is so polite and respectful, everyone who gets to know him loves him. His courteousness serves him well and helps solidify his relationships.

Sometimes we have to go above and beyond society's expectations to ensure that our kids have a good quality of life. I put an emphasis on teaching David manners because I know that his speech and social skills are delayed. I want him to make friends and maintain employment, but without having conversational language skills and the ability to socialize in a typical fashion, that can be difficult.

As our kids transition into adolescence and adulthood, there are steps we can take to help them be successful. The Essential Life Skills chart may be a tad intimidating but imagine how intimidating those tasks would be if our children waited to learn all of those skills as an adult. Most disability resource centers are well equipped to help parents during this transition; they have entire departments for adult transitional services and can provide you with lists for first aid classes, safety skills, money management, and other life skills.

If your disability resource center is not particularly helpful, your child's middle and high-school teachers and support staff should have some creative ideas as to how to address the transition to adulthood. Transition services should be added to the IEP in eleventh grade and you can help establish goals for transition services. As with all things pertaining to autism, we often need advice from the experts. If you aren't impressed with the available resources at your disability resource center or child's school, you always have the option of adding these skills to your child's therapy goals.

WORK ON SAFETY SKILLS

In terms of essential life skills, the most critical and important skill set we can teach is **safety**. Many children with autism do not have adequate safety-awareness skills, and as they grow into adults, the need to enhance these skills increases exponentially. If there is only one life skill we teach our kids, it should be swimming. I know that sounds crazy. We see swimming as a recreational activity, but for people with autism swimming is an essential, potentially lifesaving skill.

It's heartbreaking, but the truth is that wandering is the leading cause of death for people with autism. Of those deaths, 90% are caused by drowning. Learning to swim is a necessity for people with autism. Some rec centers or therapy centers host special-needs swim classes. If you are looking for classes in your area, your best bet is to reach out to your local Autism Society or Parent to Parent and ask if there are special-needs swim classes in your area.

When David was little I put him in swim classes every year for four years. We did one lesson with a one-on-one instructor, and although he learned to hold his breath and tread water, he did not learn to swim from any of the classes I enrolled him in over the course of those four years.

Several years ago, a little girl with autism drowned not far from my house. I was plagued by it. I couldn't sleep well for days after she passed away. I would stay up thinking about the places David would go if he wandered, and instinctively I knew he would head to a local pool or nearby lake. I knew that the only way I could ever sleep well again is if I taught him to swim.

I spent the next few months teaching him how to swim by myself. I took him to the pool by my house almost every day for two months. I bought a bag of inexpensive toys, and every time he'd swim on his own, I would give him a prize. By the end of the summer, he was able to swim the length of the pool unassisted. Once he had mastered swimming, I was able to sleep through the night again.

Wandering is a serious issue in our community, and although I will cover it in greater detail in chapter eight, the best thing we can do is teach our kids how to swim as an essential life skill. It may be one of the most important things we can do as the parent of a child with autism.

Safety skills are going to look different for each child on the spectrum. In our case, David is terrible about looking both ways before crossing the street, and he's even worse in parking lots. Despite my best efforts, he is still not able to cross a street or even walk in a parking lot by himself.

I have added both of these to his behavioral therapy goals. His BCBA takes him on walks, and they practice crossing the street over and over again. They also walk through parking lots near our home to get David used to looking for cars that are backing out of or pulling into spaces where he is walking. Although David is now looking for cars when crossing the street or walking in a parking lot, he doesn't always stop when he sees the car coming. It's maddening.

It's a never-ending battle to get him to grasp basic safety concepts. Recently we went to Target and he started to walk away from me when we were in the parking lot. I called him back. Had he kept going, a big SUV would have backed right into him. At this point I had to pull out the big guns to get him to understand safety in parking lots and while crossing the street—I took away his Kindle (gasp!). It's the most severe punishment I can dole out. He loves his Kindle more than any other earthly possession. It's his way to listen to his beloved Adele and watch YouTube videos of Super Mario Bros. Although I hate to take away his favorite thing, it is the surest way to get his attention.

In terms of safety skills, it's also important to have a conversation about physical boundaries and explain what is, and is not, appropriate touch. We also need to talk to our kids about what a healthy relationship looks like and what being taken advantage of looks like. In line with their inability to read social cues, they may miss red flags if a person is trying to deceive or manipulate them.

As our kids enter adulthood, we have to consider their vulnerability and start to make arrangements for **guardianship** if needed. If your child is considered disabled, you will need to establish guardianship when they turn eighteen. Autism and guardianship are tricky. Some of our kids can make their own decisions and do not need a guardian, while others will need to be protected by a guardian for the rest of their life.

Guardianship is determined by the courts. People with autism who can live independently, work, and pay their own bills do not need a guardian but may require a representative to ensure they are not being taken advantage of financially. On the other hand, if a person with autism cannot care for themselves, cannot manage money, and cannot get to doctor's appointments on their own, they will need a guardian and a financial representative (one person can act as both).

If an adult with autism needs a guardian, the courts will usually assign the role to the parents or adult siblings. If there are no immediate family members available, a friend of the family can act as guardian. If friends are not able to serve as guardian, the courts assign a professional guardian who oversees finances and day-to-day care.

Many of us do not have a long list of people we can trust to care for our child when we no longer can. Because it can be difficult to find caregivers, it is important that we start to think about who we want to care for our kids if we fall ill or pass away. I will cover special needs trusts in chapter 9, but for now it's imperative that we start to think critically about who a legal guardian for our child can be. Many special needs trusts will ask you to list at least five people who can care for your child when you no longer can. As our kids age into adulthood, guardianship becomes one of the most critical issues we face as parents. It is a good idea to begin thinking about what your child will need in adulthood and to start financial and possible long-term planning early.

If your child needs a guardian, when he transitions to adult services, the guardian becomes responsible for keeping up with therapy, doctors' visits and even grocery shopping. Adult services offered through your disability resource center will include a service plan. That service plan can include behavioral therapy to teach safety awareness, money management, and other life skills. The transition into adult services can be a bit jarring for families. Medicaid waivers and private insurance fund treatment and therapy in order to help a person with a disability gain independent living skills. If a person with a disability is not independent by adulthood, funding becomes limited when adult service programs kick in. Adult services and waivers are very limited in most states.

As our kids enter adulthood, we must give serious thought as to how they will manage when they are on their own. If a child on the spectrum can be taught adequate safety and essential life skills, the best thing we can do is pull out all the stops to make sure he is well prepared for the complexities of adulthood. If a child on the spectrum will not be able to manage their own affairs and you feel he can easily be taken advantage of, you will want to begin the process of becoming your child's guardian. Establishing guardianship requires letters from the child's doctors and therapists and may require school records. You will want to start this process about a year before your child's eighteenth birthday to ensure all of the necessary paper-work is completed in time.

TEACH BASIC HOME REPAIRS

I don't think we need to teach our kids how to build an entire house (unless they want to). However, if they are capable, teaching them how to fix little things around the house will help them save money and help them to maintain their own home.

There are simple fixes for common issues we all run into when living on our own. These things can be taught at home and can be written down so when your child is on his own, he has a source of reference if something breaks around the house.

Resetting a tripped circuit breaker is simple but needs to be taught. It occurred to me recently that David wouldn't know what to do if the breaker was tripped. For example, I have to plug my exterior Christmas lights into the same outlet as my microwave. If I forget and plug them both in at the same time, it trips the breaker and I have to reset it. The last time I did this, I showed David where the breaker box was and showed him what a tripped breaker looks like and how to turn it back on. This way when he lives on his own, he'll know what to do in this instance and won't need to call a repair person. It's something we as adults know how to do but may not think to teach our kids.

Access to fire extinguisher. Whether our kids live independently or at home with us, it's important to have a fire extinguisher handy. Fire extinguishers come with instructions, and as long as we show our kids where it is and how to use it, they can protect themselves and their home in case of a small fire. It is also important to have a conversation about what to do in case of a fire. If it's a small fire in a pan in the kitchen, a fire extinguisher may put the fire out, but in case of a grease fire, they need to know to put flour on the fire. In case of a big fire, they need to have an exit plan and know not to try and put it out themselves. Fire safety is something that must be taught because, after all, how would they know what to do if we don't tell them? Fire stations in my area host safety events, and some schools or disability resource centers partner with fire departments to address this issue. If there are fire safety courses available in your area, it is a good use of time to attend these events.

Replacing batteries in smoke alarms and carbon monoxide detectors is actually very simple, but again, if we don't teach our kids how to do it, how will they know? In my house one alarm can be reached without a ladder and the other two require a small stepladder. I have shown David how to safely use the ladder and check for corroded batteries. Teaching these simple fixes will boost self-esteem and allow for more independence.

Turning off outside water is crucial in cold-weather states. Here in Colorado, when the first freeze comes, I have to shut off my outside water line to prevent my pipes from freezing. The water-line valve is easy to switch off, and teaching David how was as simple as showing him one time. It's simple and can potentially save thousands of dollars in unnecessary repairs.

Turning off water to a leaking toilet is easy, but if a person doesn't know how to do it, they can't remedy the problem themselves. Pointing out where the shut-off valve is on the toilet and taking turns turning the valve off and on may be all you need to do to prevent costly water damage to the home.

Teaching basic home repairs does not have to be taught by an expert in most cases. If your child is capable of doing these things for himself, it will only benefit him in the long run. As your child matures it may help to keep a running list of teachable, simple home repairs. If your child can live independently, I recommend making a list, with pictures or diagrams if needed, of simple repairs as a reference if something needs fixing around the house.

PREPARE YOUR CHILD FOR PUBERTY

Puberty is a tough transition for all kids. I remember my middle-school years being some of the most awkward years of my life. For kids with autism, puberty can be especially difficult because they often can't express how they feel about the changes happening in their body. It's important that we explain to them how puberty will impact their mood and hormones.

Keep in mind, migraine headaches and seizures can start in puberty, so it's critical that our kids be able to communicate their health needs on some level. If a child in nonverbal and does not communicate, keep an eye out for signs of headaches and absence seizures. If headaches start in puberty, adding magnesium and encouraging your child to drink plenty of water may help alleviate headache pain. If your child starts to have seizures in puberty, there is the possibility that the seizures are triggered by an autoimmune response and can be addressed by building the body up.[6] About one-fourth of children with autism start to have seizures in puberty.[7]

The issue with seizures is that it's hard for doctors to pinpoint why a child starts having seizures, and therefore they aren't always sure how to treat them. If your child has seizures, you will surely end up seeing a neurologist and multiple physicians or specialists. During this process it's important to remember that most of our kids have underlying medical conditions, including autoimmunity, and nutritional and/or neurotransmitter deficiencies. Although your doctors will want to treat the seizures with medication, it's important for you to be a part of this process; you can help determine how the seizures will be addressed.

If you and your child's doctors decide anti-seizure medication is necessary, don't feel like that is your only option. Treating the underlying medical conditions and building up the immune system should be factored into your child's seizure plan. Here in Colorado I have met several people who moved here specifically to treat their child's seizures with CBD oil, cannabidiol, a non-psychoactive marijuana derivative. Although seizures are scary, they can be treated; how you will treat them will be determined by yourself and the physicians who work with your child. Our lives have been so damaged by pharmaceutical companies that it's hard for me to trust their products. If David started having seizures again, I would detox him as seizures are the number-one reported vaccine injury and have his immune system checked out. I'd use camels' milk and CBD, but after all we've been through, I see meds as a last resort.

However, some seizures must be treated with medication. There are things you can do to limit the amount of seizure meds your child takes. Finding a physician who understands the importance of treating underlying medical conditions in children with autism is a must. My dad's seizures are somewhat under control with the use of meds, but when I suggested adding magnesium to help decrease seizure activity, the doctor looked at me like I had two heads. I explained that magnesium helps to regulate the central nervous system and that it is needed for neurotransmitter production. The doctor rolled his eyes and dismissed the possibility that magnesium could potentially decrease seizure activity.

The point is, seizures often decrease as magnesium intake is increased. Working with a doctor who applies common sense and reason to treating seizure disorders is best. According to epilepsy.com "Low magnesium levels can lead to seizures and also can cause low calcium levels."[8] The fact that many doctors ignore vitamins, supplements, and diet as a way to increase health and boost the immune system is beyond my comprehension. I have been told by every doctor who sees David, "The diet won't work. It's just a waste of money." Yet those same doctors marvel at his progress and send parents of kids with autism to *me* for advice. Point being, there are times when doctors have limited solutions to complex medical issues. Sometimes thinking outside the box and trying new strategies is more beneficial than continuing treatments and drugs that aren't curing the body. Western medicine tends to treat health problems with prescription drugs. While drugs may mitigate symptoms, they rarely cure a disease or disorder. In my mind, mitigating symptoms is a temporary fix, and while seizure meds may be necessary in the short term, magnesium, a clean diet, CBD, and detox can help stop (or decrease) seizure activity in the long term. Always keep an open mind about treatment; your input matters, and you should never feel bad about having a say in your child's health. Your voice matters when it comes to determining medical treatments for your child.

Puberty is an interesting time of life. David, who is well behaved 99% of the time, has started giving me dirty looks and will occasionally throw himself on the floor in an act of defiance against bedtime. He can be happy, then grumpy, then happy again. Then he's sad, then he's happy, then he's bored, then he's grumpy, then he's happy—all this, in the span of one hour. The hormonal fluctuations are tough, and they can present themselves differently from one minute to the next. Although it's not always fun, it's possible to take the emotional roller coaster in stride and simply ignore the majority of their outbursts and dirty looks. It isn't personal; they are in the awkward teenage years and are experiencing hormonal fluctuations and, most likely, wanting to hang out with kids their age and do typical teenage activities. These years are tough on typical kids but even harder on kids with autism. They need our time, patience, and love more than ever during these years.

When talking to our kids about puberty, it's important to let them know what to expect. Explaining to our kids that they are growing and their body is changing is important. When we take the time to explain what changes in hormones makes us feel like, it can help ease their anxiety when they start to feel sudden changes in emotions but don't understand why.

As parents we don't always know how to address an issue. Puberty for kids on the spectrum can be tough, especially for those kids who have little-to-no communication abilities. If you feel like your child is having a difficult time during puberty, there is always the option of using essential oils. Geranium, lavender, and rose essential oils seem to be the most commonly used oils for puberty. Although they are not a cure-all, these oils can help kids feel centered and calm.

TACA has excellent resources, links, books, and articles on their website pertaining to puberty. If you are looking for more information, it is a great place to start.[9] Personally, I was not prepared for David hitting puberty. Since he started feeling better, he's always been a happy little guy. Now that he's hit puberty, he's still happy but definitely more moody and more likely to throw himself on the ground out of frustration. David says, "Where are my friends? When will I do my first stuff like the movies and sleepovers with my friends?" Not only is he experiencing hormonal and emotional changes, he is also becoming more aware of the fact that he is missing out on social activities with his peers. It's got to be tough on him, and the best I can do is love him, tell him how great he is, and remind him that this is a normal part of growing up. Sometimes the best thing we can do is love them through the hard times (even when they roll their eyes at us).

When it comes to talking about sex and masturbation, I am not the expert. I am going to buy one of the books

THE AUTISM HELP BOOK

recommended by TACA and deal with it that way. My mom is Catholic and very conservative about certain things. She never had "the talk" with me, and honestly, I have no idea how to talk to my son about this subject. I have talked to David about safety and not letting anyone touch him inappropriately, but the sex talk has not yet occurred. As much as we don't want to talk to our kids about sex, we have to. We have to talk about boundaries, consent, personal space, love, marriage, abuse, all of it. We have to have this conversation with our kids. *How* you have that conversation is up to you. We all have our own personal and religious beliefs. How we approach this subject is personal, and it is up to you to decide how you will address sexuality.

Having autism does not mean sexual development is delayed. Although some people with autism may not express a desire to have sex, many people on the spectrum do want to have intimate relationships. Even if your child appears to have no interest in sex, talking about boundaries and not letting people touch their privates is necessary. Again, the ability to communicate is critical; find some way your child can communicate and hurtful or inappropriate interactions with others. I hate to be a downer, but nonverbal children are far more likely to be abused than verbal children. Communication, is not an option; it is a necessity. Even if your child only learns two words in sign language, yes and no, you will have a way to communicate about their experiences.

If your child indicates he or she wants to have sex, selecting one of the books from the TACA website may help, or you can address it in your own way. We don't have to give the perfect talk. We simply need to have "the talk" at some point during their teenage years.[10]

Girls who have autism need different things than boys during puberty. First, someone has to talk to them about their period and how to address it. Second, we live in a society in which women are objectified on a regular basis.

My sons are offended by what women wear on TV and how women are spoken about. If my boys get that women are objectified by the media, how must a girl feel? If a neurotypical teenaged girl is having a hard time finding her power in this world, where does that leave a teenaged girl who has autism? Females who have autism need extra protection and probably behavior therapy to help them learn healthy and appropriate boundaries.

Whether your child is a girl or a boy, whether verbal or nonverbal, whatever the circumstances are, sexuality must be addressed during these already awkward years.

As our children enter adolescence and adulthood, we must take the necessary steps to ensure they have a happy, safe, and fulfilling adult life whether they function at a high or low level. We will work on communication to ensure they have the ability to communicate their needs. We will work with them, their therapists, and their school to teach essential life skills. We will strive to teach safety skills and basic home repairs and help them understand their changing body.

As our children enter adulthood, a new set of challenges presents itself. The best thing we can do for our children is prepare them for adulthood, whether that means establishing guardianship or teaching them independent living skills. As they mature their needs change, as does society's expectations of them. In preparing our children for the adult world, the goal is always to build up their self-esteem and fine tune their skill set to help them successfully transition into adulthood.

NOTES FOR CHAPTER 7

8

YOUR NEW LIFE

What lies behind us and what lies ahead of us
are tiny matters compared to what lies within us.

—Henry David Thoreau

IN WRITING THIS CHAPTER, I am made to think about the
hard times: David's constant screaming; the ugly stares of
strangers; my feelings of loneliness and isolation. Those days
are now my past (beside the occasional ugly stares of strangers). I decided years ago that I would not concede, I would
not surrender, I would not wave the white flag, and I haven't.
I *refused* to cave into negativity and rejected the belief that
my son could not recover. Today our life is a life restored.
We got here by my will and my absolute refusal to give up on
the prospect of us having a happy, fulfilling life. Your life, as
impossible as it may seem today, can be restored.

Thriving in the midst of hardship is possible. For me
the key has been visualization and the belief that things will
turn around for the better. This may sound odd, but years
ago I had a dream about David, and I have held that dream
in my heart and in my mind as if it were real. It has carried
me through many bad days.

In my dream, David was eighteen and a senior in high
school. He walked into my parents' kitchen and spoke to
me as if he never had autism. I burst into tears and said, "I

can't believe you're okay. I knew this day would come. I just can't believe how far you've come." David looked at me and said, "Mom I'm fine. But really, I'm going to be fine, Mom."

Although it was just a dream, I have held onto that image: the image of my son speaking to me in sentences, the image of him about to graduate from high school, the image of him as a healthy, capable young man. I have held onto that image of my son being healthy and our lives restored. As the years go by, he gets better and better, and that dream is close to becoming a reality. Believing things will get better is the first and most important step in reclaiming your life.

It is the mind that determines our path, not money, not education, not social status, but the mind that dictates where we will go and how successful we will be (although having tons of money and a good home could make life easier). When our child is diagnosed with autism, it will not be external forces that determine the success of our family but, instead, the thoughts we allocate to our lives. I started out being docile, soft-spoken, and easily intimidated. Now I speak my mind, I'm assertive, and in metaphoric terms, I take no prisoners.

Who we were before autism entered our lives and who we eventually become are two very different people. Accepting that our lives are forever changed is a necessary step in moving forward and moving past the grief. This chapter focuses on our changing lives, on accepting what is in front of us, and loving our crazy, unconventional lives.

In this chapter we will look at the ways in which our lives have changed and how to make the best of what is:

- The evolution of our relationships
- The fun of going in public
- Taking a new approach to holidays and vacations
- Maintaining our own health
- Restoring peace of mind—addressing autism and wandering

THE EVOLUTION OF OUR RELATIONSHIPS

When I realized David had autism, I knew that my life would be permanently changed. Little did I know that my social life would be permanently changed as well. As time went on we were invited to fewer events, fewer parties, and fewer play dates, until one day I realized we weren't being invited to much at all.

David's behavior was severe and uncontrollable. I suppose us being left out of events wasn't personal but merely practical. After all, David did have a tendency to tear down decorations and the probability of him attacking party guests and throwing birthday cake was exponentially high. I get why we weren't invited to things anymore, but what hurt me was the absence of certain people altogether. Even though we couldn't go anywhere without a cataclysmic meltdown, I still needed friends, support, and a sense of community. The realization that many of the people around me were fair-weather friends was difficult to accept and an unneeded blow to my already-bruised ego.

Fake people, bad people, people with an agenda, people who love us only conditionally have seen themselves out of our lives. Those who truly love us unconditionally have stayed by our side, and those people are my tribe. If the people around you are dropping like flies, they are not your tribe. In time you will find your people, the tribe of people who love you, your child, and your crazy life. There is only one way I can accurately explain this critical concept: David is my bullshit detector.

When I went to a TACA conference recently, I felt as if I had found my tribe of warrior mothers. I have had the same friends since I was a kid, and I love and cherish my friendships with them, but at some point, I realized that I needed to find my autism mom peeps. Meeting other parents from

TACA was a life-changing experience for me. They got me. They get why I spend more money on food than my mortgage. They get why I skip vacations and fancy clothes in order to fund David's out-of-pocket care. They get why I am scared of tap water and why I stop my life to fight bad legislation when it comes up in my state. They get me, and I get them. The goal is always to make and keep friends who will build you up and be part of your support system. Autism, if nothing else, will weed out the people in our lives who are not truly invested in us and our future.

Wherever your people are, wherever your tribe can be found, is the objective: find support and a sense of community. In some states, local Autism Societies offer family events. TACA has chapters in most states, and Parent to Parent is a good way to connect with local moms and dads. It may take time, but eventually, you will start to make friends who not only get your life but who can help improve it as well.

If I learned anything about how having a child with autism impacts friendships, it is that your real friends will stand by you under any circumstances. The time I spent agonizing over missed parties and checking the mail for invitations that would never come was wasted time. Anyone who isn't meant to be in your life and who isn't your real friend will either leave or make it clear they are not invested in your child nor the betterment of your life. Some people see themselves out of our lives, and some people need to be shown the door. Either way, the sooner we eliminate negative people from our lives, the sooner we'll have time to get out and track down our tribe. Finding your people, the people who make your life better and accept you as you are, is liberating. With time and persistence, you will find your tribe.

Friendships are important; they allow us to be ourselves and to open up without fear of rejection. Marriage is hugely important too. Marriage can be tough under the best of circumstances, but when we add the stress of caring for a child who has autism and often other underlying medical conditions, the threads that hold our marriage together can start to fray.

After his regression, David was so severe that we literally couldn't leave him with anyone. I suppose if autism did impact our marriage, that was why. We simply didn't have time together as a couple anymore. We couldn't go out to dinner, go to a movie, go to a friend's house, nothing; we had no time together outside of the home. In addition to that, things fell apart for us for a million other reasons, and in my case, we would have gotten divorced even if David hadn't had autism. We faced odds that no couple could overcome, and David had no bearing on that aspect of our lives. Things just fell apart, and although autism added to the pressure we faced, it was not a deciding factor in our divorce.

The words we speak to our spouses are very powerful. When I was married I stayed home with David and had no one to talk to all day. My ex worked two jobs most of the time in order for me to finish college and so we could pay for David's mounting medical bills. When he came home from working two jobs, I often dumped on him the minute he walked in the door. I told him about everything that went wrong that day, all of the things I was worried about, and every potential impending catastrophe that I had dreamed up while he was busy working. Basically, this poor guy worked two jobs to support us and instead of getting an "I love you; glad you're home," he walked into a complaint-fest on many occasions. Point being, yes, we're stressed and, yes, autism can be hard, but it's hard on our spouses too. Taking inventory of every good thing your spouse contributes to the household can go a long way in maintaining a healthy marriage. When we speak words of gratitude and love over our spouse, our marriage can heal from old wounds and gain roots.

Although I am no expert in marriage, I know I could have done some things differently and certainly better. If I could go back, I would have told him how much I appreciated his hard work and dedication to his family more often and I would have complained less.

For me, staying home with kids is harder than the years I worked and went to school. Parenting is a day-and-night job with few breaks and no pay. The only thanks we get may be from our spouse, and while we may rock yoga pants every day, have crazy hair, and unidentifiable stains on our clothes, we still need to hear that what we're doing is valuable and that we look amazing. Marriage is not easy, but it isn't necessarily as hard as we make it out to be either. Adding in a few compliments and the occasional dinner sans kids could make all the difference to a struggling marriage.

Although I think people should always try to save their marriage, that isn't always a possibility. Adultery, abuse, and substance abuse are deal breakers in many marriages. In some instances, the best and healthiest thing to do is walk away. Divorce is hard on kids and can be particularly hard on kids with autism. Our kids generally have few friends and little social interaction, the family unit is immensely important to them. If your marriage is unsalvageable and you decide to divorce, your child with autism will need special attention and most likely some form of therapy to heal.

TACA has a great link on divorce.[1] As it pertains to children with autism, divorce can be a complex matter. We need to determine parenting time, establish a special needs trust, and fund the trust after the divorce. We need to discuss who pays for therapy, extracurricular activities, and the like. The link provided in the endnotes is a good place to start when ironing out the details.

Several months after my ex and I split, I started dating Brooks' father. The red flags were there: We only saw each other at night (the only time I had a babysitter). There were times when I couldn't reach him and he wouldn't respond to my texts. He didn't seem very interested in my interests, and we often met at a place called El Diablo. The signs were there, and I ignored them.

When I found out I was pregnant with Brooks, I immediately told his dad. We had been dating for eight months at that point, and to my knowledge we were monogamous. I was wrong. Long story short, we tried to make it work— we both love Brooks so much and wanted him to grow up with two parents in the home— but there were barrages of issues. For what it's worth, Brooks got many good qualities from his dad. Brooks is a talented artist, smart, and strong willed. Despite the less-than-ideal circumstances with his father and I, I love my little Brooks and appreciate the joy he brings into our lives.

If I learned anything it's that, as an autism mama, I either need to date the right guys or not at all. We all have our own baggage, and the reality is I never dealt with mine. I was young when I had David, and it's been a whirlwind ever since. I have never, until recently, taken the time to address my own needs and unpack some of my baggage. In terms of dating I feel like I need to work on myself for a while before I jump into anything. The most important thing to me (and probably you too) is my children. For the sake of our kids and ourselves, it is best to take time and heal before we enter the dating world.

As autism parents we often get mistreated in public, by our families, by fair-weather friends, by insurance companies, by school staff, by doctors, etc. When a person has grown accustomed to being mistreated, it becomes normal. In terms of dating the best thing we can do is stay single long enough to get healthy emotionally, physically, and spiritually so we are in a place to make critical decisions like choosing a partner. To me the most important thing would be finding a man who will be good to my children. Until I find a warrior tough enough to hang with my feisty self and three strong-willed boys, I'm better off being single. Now that I have taken time to get healthy, get back in church, read self-help books, and go to therapy, I know that no relationship is better than a bad relationship.

Autism changes everything. It changes the dynamics of our friendships, our marriage, and even sometimes the dynamics of our familial relationships. Family is important, and sometimes the best way to maintain a bond with our family is to be honest. I have gotten to the point that before going to a family gathering, I will send out little information sheets on autism. I also list helpful tips for interacting with David and list his interests, so they have something to talk about with him. I explain what sensory overload feels like and how to avoid it. I explain what autism feels like to him and that his autism and inability to socialize in a typical fashion are isolating to him. He does not want to be isolated, but if he is overwhelmed by sensory input, his autism will force him into isolation and he will go to a quiet room or ask to wait in the car.

My family means well and truly wants to interact with David and make him feel welcome. Before I started sending out autism information sheets to family, the interaction between them and David was limited and somewhat uncomfortable. After I started sending out the information sheets, everything changed. Family gatherings became an enjoyable experience because my family knew to avoid tons of sensory stimuli like loud music and touching. Once they knew that peanuts, wheat, dairy, and soy were not on his diet, they started making things he could eat.

Family is important, and when the relationships with our family are strained, it makes life harder on us. Sometimes the best way to help build the relationship between our family and our child with autism is simply with a little information. If family relationships are strained following the diagnosis, it can't hurt to reach out to people and provide some helpful tips for interacting with our kids. As a mother I am very protective of David and very sensitive to how people treat him. He is kind, gentle, and always good. As far as I'm concerned, he is the perfect child. Because I am fiercely protective of him, I have found that being proactive and addressing his autism before family gatherings can help to avoid hard feelings and misunderstandings.

As an autism mama I will admit I can be a bit of a martyr. When I can I buy my kids nice clothes, shoes, coats, take them on adventures, pay for any activities they want to do and provide them with the best (often expensive) food money can buy. I do so much for my kids that I have to remind myself to do things for myself once in a while.

As time goes by asking for and accepting help here and there has become a little easier. Some of you may have family that don't understand or respect you. In these cases setting boundaries and taking a step back from the relationship may be in order. If, however, you have a supportive family but feel overwhelmed by the stress of raising a child with autism, it may be time to ask for a little help.

In an article titled "9 Ways You Can Support a Special Needs Parent," writer M. Lin eloquently explains what we need from the people who love us:

> **Insist on helping**. No matter how "together" I appear on the outside, I can always use help. In fact, sometimes appearing "together" is the only way I can make it through the day myself. You'll notice I didn't write "offer to help."

She goes on to say:

> **Ask me how I'm doing**. My friends often ask me about Jacob...which I love, but it would also be nice if occasionally they asked me about how I'm doing —not in my career, or my hobbies or dating life, but how I'm doing in this role as a special needs parent. I don't often get to talk about how hard it can be, or how I'm tired, or how I had a good day or bad day. It might just be me, but a sincere "How are you doing handling everything?" once in

a while, and readiness to hear an honest answer is all I need to feel like someone cares.[2]

This writer expresses what we all feel but often don't share with the people in our lives. Maybe our family does want to support us, but they just don't know how. Maybe they do worry about us, our kids, and our health but don't want to overstep their boundaries by saying so. Maybe the best way to bridge that gap is to start a conversation about the type of support you need. I personally find it difficult to talk about how hard life is as a single mom without crying, so for me handing family an article like the one above or sharing it on social media is the best way for me to address it. I am not comfortable asking for help, but I also know I can't do this alone. Letting the people in my life know that I need and appreciate their support has been liberating for me.

Letting my guard down and being honest about how hard my life is has opened up the doors of communication between me and my family. Being honest about our lives allows the people who love us to offer support in the ways they can. If you aren't comfortable asking for help outright, giving someone a physical copy of an article that resonates with you will allow them to read it more than once, and they can revisit it now and again.

Maintaining relationships with our families can be more challenging than one would expect. If and when we're faced with these challenges, it's important to address them as quickly as possible. If someone upsets me, I have what I call a three-day rule. I am so touchy about David that when things happen with him, my first reaction is come to his defense and turn into a lioness. However, if I give myself a few days to calm down before I respond to someone who has offended me or David, it allows me to come up with solutions rather than criticisms (which never get a person very far). Educating our families on autism and how to interact with our kids can be as simple as handing them an article or sitting down and talking to them about the kind of support we need. I believe it's best to give family a chance to correct their behavior before cutting them off; after all, our kids need all the support and love they can get.

In terms of relationships, possibly the hardest relationship there is to care for is the relationship we have with our typical children. When David was two, I had Aidan. A year later their dad and I divorced. I went back to work, and David and Aidan spent nine hours a day with babysitters or in a day care. When I was home, most of my attention went to David. David was completely falling apart when he was three, and there was my little baby Aidan—cute, chubby, happy Aidan. I compensated for the lost time with him by taking breaks from David to hold him, squeeze him, and carry him in my arms until they were too tired to carry him. I knew Aidan was missing out on my attention, and the only way I could compensate was to make sure that every day he had as many hugs and kisses as I could work in. It was the best I could do.

As years went by I worked, did research on autism, took David to therapy several times a week, and kept up with his blood draws, doctors' appointments and IEPs; there was little time to focus on Aidan. When David started getting better around age four, I made it a point to take Aidan to swim class, the park or baby gym. I went out of my way to have time with just him and me whenever possible. I volunteered at his school when I could. I go to every soccer practice and game and try to make time for him to do the things he enjoys.

The reality is that, although I tried to be attentive to him, Aidan missed out on a lot of his childhood while I took care of David. I wish that weren't the case, but it is. Aidan missed out on time at the park and time playing with his mom while I fought with insurance companies, cleaned up after David and sat through David's therapies. Aidan missed out on so much, and yet he is positive, kind, loving, generous, funny, and an all-around great kid. Recently, I said, "Aidan I'm sorry. I feel like you have missed out on so much while I took care of David. I'll try to make it up to you." Aidan replied, "What are you talking about Mom? He's my brother. You had to do that so he could get better. You had to save his life. Don't ever say that again. He needed you more than I did." And there it is, proof positive that, in spite of the obstacles, I have raised a nice, hardheaded, and compassionate young man.

Although Aidan has no hard feelings toward his brother, that is not always the case when it comes to siblings. In life, almost nothing is black and white, but when it comes to the matter of siblings of children with developmental delays, it seems to be a very black-and-white matter. Either the typical sibling is loving and supportive or they are hurt and resentful. In my personal experience, there isn't much grey area when it comes to siblings.

If a typical child is struggling with resentment toward his or her sibling, I think it's good for them to have an opportunity to talk about it without judgment. In many cases, their lives are harder because their sibling has autism, and maybe all they need is for a parent or adult to acknowledge how difficult it is. If a typical child has sacrificed sports, sleepovers with friends, vacations, time with his or her parents, it's important that at some point, an adult acknowledge that sacrifice. In truth, most siblings who act out are doing so because they are hurt. They hurt when they see their parents struggle. They hurt when they miss another event because their sibling with autism is having a meltdown. They hurt when they are always second. The pain siblings feel is valid and understandable. Giving a sibling an extra compliment each day and spending one-on-one time here and there can be life-changing for them.

THE FUN OF GOING IN PUBLIC

If you have a super well-behaved child with autism, feel free to skip this section. If, however, you have a child with autism who struggles with public outings, much of this will resonate with you. When David was violent and having regular meltdowns, going out in public was nearly impossible. Trips to the store often ended in colossal tantrums, with people staring and David hitting me and himself. It was awful.

It got to the point that I was staying home all the time. I didn't socialize at all, and the only time I ever got out of the house (besides going to work) was to go to the store, which was nearly impossible given his behavior. When we did go into a store, he would pick a toy and throw a screaming fit, complete with throwing himself on the floor, if I did not buy the toy he wanted. After one particularly bad trip to Target, I decided I had had enough and was going to modify his behavior. If the only way I could get out of the house was to take him with me, I had to find a way to manage his behavior.

I decided that the best way to modify his behavior was essentially to "set him up." I asked my parents to watch Aidan, and I took David to Target. I knew David would pick out a toy and would melt down when I refused to buy it. He went straight to the toy aisle and picked out a very expensive Lego set. I said, "Mommy will buy you special presents on your birthday and Christmas, but today we are not buying that." As we walked around the store, I reminded him that I would not be buying his toy and that I needed to put it back. The second he started to have a tantrum I took him out of the store.

I did this every weekend for six weeks. I would take him in there, and if he refused to put his toy down or if he threw a fit, I picked him up and took him to the car. He learned that if he misbehaved, he would have to leave. By the seventh week, we went into Target and were able to leave without the toy he had chosen, and he didn't throw a fit, scream or hit me.

In terms of behavior modification, our kids need to learn that for every action there is a reaction. If we cave every time they throw a fit, their behavior will never improve. Sometimes it takes demonstrating, in real time, the consequences of negative behaviors. As David's behaviors improved we were able to go to more places, and it benefited the whole family. He, Aidan, and I would go shopping almost every weekend to give us something to do. In time, David understood that if he behaved in the store, he could get something small like a toy car or candy and that was enough to keep him happy. If he did misbehave, I left my cart and immediately took him to the car. It wasn't ideal, but I knew that I had to help him understand that there are consequences for negative behavior and that I would not reward him for misbehaving.

David was little when I modified his behavior and I know that it is more difficult as children get older. When our kids are little, we can pick them up and carry them to the car. If they are teenagers and weigh more than we do, that's a different story. When older kids misbehave in public, addressing the behavior can be very challenging. If you feel that public outings are overly difficult, you can seek out the advice of a behavior specialist and possibly an OT if you think the issue is related to sensory stimuli. Some therapy centers allow their employees to go out in public with clients, if you have an opportunity to go in public with your child's behavior therapist, I would recommend doing so. If your behavior therapist is not able to go in public with you, write down possible triggers for your child's behavior and specific behaviors you see while in public. Your therapist should be able to help you come up with creative solutions to modify behavior.

In some cases, negative behaviors can be attributed to sensory issues. Fluorescent lights, for example, used to throw David into frenzy. He didn't deal well with large crowds, loud music, or too much noise. If sensory sensitivity is the driving force behind public outbursts, try to address the sensory piece before your next outing. If your child is particularly sensitive to sound, noise-blocking headphones work wonders. If too much noise or crowds are the problem, implementing the Wilbargar Brushing Technique or using a weighted vest or fidget toy may work wonders.

Then there is the ever-present, unwelcome issue of people staring at us in public. This is something we must all deal with in our own way. I decided it was perhaps best to start ignoring people in public after I yelled at a lady at T.J. Maxx. On that particular day, I was very proud of David for how he handled himself in the store; he was doing his best to stay close to me in line. He wasn't misbehaving, he wasn't yelling, and he wasn't trying to run away; it was a huge improvement from where we started. He was stimming by flapping his hands and making noises, but he was not being bad in any way.

The lady behind me was staring at him and giving me dirty looks. I ignored her until she snidely said, "What a great kid. Nice parenting." I, having worked all day, having driven three hours in rush-hour traffic, and being on my period (sorry, guys, but it's the truth) was not having any of that. I turned around and said, "Look. He has had intensive therapy since he was two. This is a huge improvement. He has autism. He can't help it, but you, however, can help how you treat people. His dad is gone, and no one will help me with him. My life is so hard most people wouldn't last a day in my shoes. Do you want to help? Do you want to babysit? Do you want to help with his medical bills? Because if not, you need to learn a lesson in manners, and next time, maybe you should suss out if a child is disabled before you insult him and his mother." The lady looked shocked and started to cry. She put her things down and hurried out of the store.

This was not my best moment, but on that day I was too tired to deal with her comments about my precious little guy. Luckily, I discovered cards from TACA that read, "My Child Is Not Misbehaving. My Child Has Autism." So now when people stare and it becomes overwhelming for me, I just hand them a card and go on with my day. No more yelling at random people in public for me.

Going in public can be fun again, but like everything else pertaining to autism, it will require some ingenuity and strategy. Public outings can be enjoyable once we find the right interventions that will work with our child.

TAKING A NEW APPROACH TO HOLIDAYS AND VACATIONS

Family gatherings are supposed to be fun and enjoyable. However, when you bring your child to a relative's house that is full of food they can't eat, when they're surrounded by people who insist on patting their head, and they are bombarded by noise and new people, the fun gets sucked right out a of family gathering.

In order to fully participate in family events, including holidays, it may be necessary to reach out to family beforehand. If it's a family picnic, for example, I will send my family texts, call them, or send a Facebook message before the picnic. I explain that David is on a special diet and ask them to please not hand him any food and to please let me feed him while we're there. I also tell them that he loves Adele, Mario Brothers, and YouTube videos so they have something to talk about with him. I share that David has a tendency to wander off and ask that they help me keep an eye on him. I do this so they start to think about ways to support me and communicate with him before we get to the picnic. It's worked out well; most people will rise to the occasion if given the opportunity to do so.

I tell people that David may not want to have a deep conversation, but he wants to be included in activities. I explain that he likes to give high-fives, he likes Frisbee, and he likes music, dancing, and cartoons. The purpose of me sharing this information with family and friends is to decrease the awkward interactions that occur when people have no background in autism. Giving our family something to work with before they interact with our kids can help facilitate the bond between our child and family. A little bit of information on autism can go a long way. Giving family and friends the tools they need to successfully engage our kids can make the holidays a great experience and can help to foster bonding.

Holidays can go smoothly when we plan well and talk to our families beforehand, but what about vacations? Most of us, including myself, don't go on vacation often. When David was little, it would have been impossible to get him on an airplane or take him on a long road trip. In those days, I longed for the fun-filled family vacations my friends were able to take. Around that time, I read the book *The Secret,* by Rhonda Burn, which helped me stay more positive and to start thinking about our lives differently. I decided that even though we couldn't go on an out-of-state vacation, we could go somewhere close to home.

Colorado has resort towns, water parks, amusement parks, wildlife preserves, and more. I decided that instead of getting upset about everything we *couldn't* do, I would find something we *could* do as a family. For several years, my ex-husband and I took the kids to Estes Park every summer. David did well in the car, and I figured the two-hour drive up there would be manageable. I reserved a hotel room that had a full kitchen so I could make his meals while we were there. I brought all of our own food to avoid infractions and made us a picnic lunch to take on our adventures during the day. I also called the hotel ahead of time to let them know my son has autism and tends to scream when excited and asked that they call me if they received complaints.

Estes Park has a ton of great family activities. They have a little amusement park for kids, a tram, fishing, boats, and

David's favorite, lots of wildlife. I called the amusement park the week before we were scheduled to come up and asked to speak to the manager; I told him the dates we would be coming and explained that my son has autism. I asked if he could speak to the staff who would be working that weekend and explain to them that he doesn't speak but understands the instructions they give him. I explained what autism is and how it affects my son, and the manager was very receptive to what I was saying.

When we went to the amusement park, I introduced myself to the manager and he said, "We've been waiting for you. Glad you're here." Then he walked us up to the big slides where the staff greeted us with smiles and excitement. The staff was patient, kind, and very accommodating while we were there. When David decided to go on the bungee-cord trampoline, the teenagers working let him take extra time, gave him high-fives, and lots of praise. A simple, five-minute conversation with the manager had made the park a joyous and fun experience for David.

We went to Estes Park for several summers, and as David got better and the behaviors decreased, we started planning our first trip out of state. Because this would be David's first trip on an airplane, I called the airline and spoke with a supervisor. The supervisor told me that the Autism Society had done training on autism and assured me her staff was fully prepared to meet his needs. When we got to security, I took my family to the front of the line, according to federal law, people with disabilities can go to the front of the line in public places if needed, and when we got to the security guards, I explained that my son had autism and that he didn't like to be touched. They gave him a high-five and stood with him while my ex and I went through security.

When we got to the plane, we were the first people on. We were the first people off the airplane as well to avoid any meltdowns (also an accommodation under the ADA). To avoid the stress David would feel in an airport, we each brought a carry-on bag so we could hurry out of there and not have to wait for luggage. This particular trip was a big deal; it was my boys' first trip to Disneyland, and David was excited beyond belief. I, of course, had called Disneyland before we left Colorado and asked which paperwork I needed to bring to demonstrate he had a federally recognized disability. When we got to Disneyland, we all went to guest services and were given bracelets that allowed us to go to the front of the line for rides.

Since that trip to Disneyland, policies have changed. Some unscrupulous people were hiring people with disabilities to accompany them to Disneyland for the sole purpose of going to the front of the lines. Although federal law under the ADA requires reasonable accommodations be made, Disneyland changed their accommodation policy to be similar to their ordinary fastpass policy. This means that while we must now wait as long as others, we don't have to do the bulk of the waiting standing in line. Waiting in line is impossible for many people with autism, and policy changes will mean many people with autism cannot go. Most of our kids don't have much of a childhood to speak of outside of therapy and doctors' visits; taking David there was my way of trying to salvage a bit of the magic of childhood. It's really too bad some thoughtless people were able to impact Disney's policies and take even more of the magic of childhood from our kids.

Whether you are taking your child on a road trip or on an airplane, communication is key. Calling the hotel, amusement park, or airline before you arrive can make a world of difference. In my experience, most people will rise to the occasion when given the opportunity to do so. In Estes Park, for example, the young men and women who worked at the amusement park were more than happy to work with David and showed him more respect and compassion than I could have imagined. With a little autism education, a vacation can be an enjoyable experience.

If you are one of the lucky people who can go on a trip without your kids, there are steps you can take to ensure your vacation is relatively stress free. I have only left my kids a few times because David's diet is complicated and food infractions can set him back significantly and I also worry about him wandering. A few months back, I attended a five-day TACA conference in California. It was the longest period of time I have ever left my kids. Before leaving, I cancelled David's therapies, made arrangements for him to be picked up from school, called his teachers to let them know I would be gone, and made sure my parents and ex-husband had a list of and access to his vitamins and supplements.

While preparing for a trip requires extra planning for parents, it is necessary that we make sure all bases are covered before leaving the state. In preparing for a trip, it's of the utmost importance that we make food and freeze it beforehand and purchase all of the food our kids can eat before we leave for vacation. Expecting grandparents and babysitters to keep them on their diet without assistance is somewhat unrealistic. Before I leave, I make David's cupcakes, brownies, and pizza and throw them in the freezer. I buy his bread, cheese, lunchmeat, mac and cheese, chips and snacks to help avoid any food infractions. I print out a food list with specific brand names just in case he runs out of things to eat while I'm away.

In addition to preplanning for the diet, many of us need to leave a list of the supplements and medications our kids take on a daily basis. David does not take medication, but he definitely needs his supplements every day. I write out what he takes and put all of his supplements in a bag or pill box so there is no confusion. In order for me to enjoy myself while I'm away from my kids, I take steps to ensure David's needs are met and he is being fed properly. It gives me peace of mind and allows me to relax while I'm away from home.

It's helpful to learn the basics of the Americans with Disabilities Act (ADA) because our kids are entitled to specific protections and accommodations when in public places. Restaurants, day care facilities, schools, etc. are required to provide reasonable accommodations for people with disabilities. Knowing the basics of the ADA can help ease the stress of planning vacations, or any public outing for that matter.[3] In short, any public entity is required by law to accommodate our children's needs, be it physical accommodations such as a wheelchair ramp or something simple like allowing a person with autism to go to the front of the line or bring their own food to a restaurant.

Holidays and vacations can still be enjoyable. We can do what everyone else does, just in a different way. As it says in *The Secret,* all good things begin in the mind. When we remain positive in our thinking, we can come up with creative ideas as to how we will address holidays and vacations. Staying positive is key to living a fulfilling life. While our lives may not be easy, we can still find the silver lining in things and devise ways to get out, socialize, and take a break once in a while.

MAINTAINING OUR OWN HEALTH

Maintaining our own health isn't always easy. We are our children's advocates, researchers, nurses, friends, and role models. In the midst of caring for our children with autism, we often forget to care for ourselves. The airplane analogy makes sense; if we are on an airplane and find ourselves in an emergency situation, we are told to put our oxygen masks on before putting them on our children. Without oxygen we will be unable to put the mask on our child. Caring for a child with autism is no different. If we want our children to thrive, we ourselves must thrive. If there is anything I have learned along the way, it's that I can't properly care for my children until and unless I care for myself.

On some level I think we all feel a bit guilty for taking time to go out with our friends, get our hair done, or go shopping. Speaking for myself, I used to feel guilty leaving David because I worried about him wandering and dietary infractions that had the potential to undermine his progress overnight. Until I got a tracker for him and felt confident that the people I left him with would keep him on his diet, I was not able to enjoy myself when I was out. It's hard to relax when our thoughts are constantly on our child's well-being.

As our child improves and safety measures are put into place, it's important that we get out of the house without the kids. Many of us take few, if any, vacations, so taking small breaks by having lunch with a friend or going to a concert becomes imperative. For several years, I didn't have any babysitters, and the only way I could get a break was to take them to the "kids' gym" at my local 24 Hour Fitness. I wouldn't say I'm big on physical fitness— I halfheartedly worked out while David and Aidan played in the kids' gym— but it gave me an hour or two to do something for myself.

Maintaining our health extends beyond taking breaks; it includes a healthy diet, too. Serotonin, which regulates mood, sleep, and appetite, is primarily made in the digestive tract. When we eat a clean, nutritious diet, our digestive tract can easily break down foods and serotonin production is properly regulated. When we eat junk food, our digestive tract can become inflamed and serotonin production is disrupted. In short, our diet directly impacts our mood.

I have been mentoring families affected by autism for over ten years, and I can say with certainty that the hardest thing for a person to do is change their (or their child's) diet. In our busy lives we don't often take time to think about what we're eating and how it will affect our health and well-being. However, the only kids I know who've recovered were on strict diets. The happiest moms I know eat well, too. There is an undeniable connection between our diet and our mental and physical well-being.

When I was thirty and diagnosed with fibromyalgia, I had two options: live with a debilitating illness or change my diet. I changed my diet, and not only did my fibromyalgia disappear, but my mood was better than ever as well. Many parents of children with autism experience physical symptoms of stress. Some parents have adrenal fatigue and are tired even after sleeping for eight hours. Some parents suffer with anxiety, while others have physical injuries from caring for their child; back injuries, for example, are common among parents of children with disabilities and many of us exhibit some physical symptoms of stress.

Anxiety and nervousness seem to impact many of us, and I know that I and several other mothers I know were able to decrease our anxiety by changing our diets. Kelly Brogan, M.D., is a holistic women's health psychiatrist who wrote the New York Times bestselling *A Mind of Your Own: The Truth about Depression and How Women Can Heal Their Bodies to Reclaim Their Lives.* She also wrote *Change Your Food, Heal Your Mood,* which you can access for free on her website.[4] Her website offers articles on gut health, depression, and motherhood. If you feel that dietary changes are in order, her website may be helpful to you.

Healthy eating has its benefits. For example, I have three kids and weigh less than I did in high school. I am happier now than ever (despite my many trials and tribulations) and feel like I finally have a handle on things. When David was at his worst, I was overwhelmed and anxious; it wasn't until I changed my diet that I noticed the impact my diet had on my mood. After I started eating mostly organic foods, my anxiety became manageable and eventually disappeared. My muscles were no longer tight, and I no longer had to diet to keep my weight down. Changing how I ate impacted both my physical and mental health.

In some instances, depression may have genetic roots, and in these cases prescription drugs may be necessary. Although some mental health conditions may require medication, most autism parents are not suffering from a genetic form of depression; our depression and anxiety is typically situational. Our situation wears us down, makes us sad, drains our finances, and can leave us isolated. Mere mortals would struggle to stay positive in our situation. If you are struggling with depression or anxiety and you and your physician do not feel it's genetic, a change in diet can greatly impact your mood and emotional stability.

Managing our health takes us back to basics. Eating well, getting exercise, and getting some sunshine and fresh air can make all the difference in the world. It's important to give yourself license to cry, grieve, and let it all out once in a while (hopefully when the kids aren't around).

As Thoreau said, "What lies behind us and what lies ahead of us are tiny matters compared to what lies within us." What lies within each one of us is the capacity to overcome the odds and whatever obstacles we face. What lies within us is the power to change our thoughts and redirect them to something positive. What lies within us is greater than what we've been through and what we're going through today. What lies within you is the ability to restore your health, your family, and your life.

RESTORING PEACE OF MIND—ADDRESSING AUTISM AND WANDERING

One of my greatest concerns with David is wandering. Worrying about him wandering off can be debilitating if I don't take the necessary steps to ensure his safety. The fact that David has had a propensity to wander means that my life is going to be a little different; how I plan vacations, his education, where he goes to summer camp, and how I address family events are all impacted by his tendency to wander.

About fifty percent of children with autism wander at some point in their lives. In addition to high incidence of wandering being reported by parents, there is the harsh reality that wandering is the leading cause of death for people with autism. Of those deaths 90% of those children drown. As I discussed in chapter 7, it is critically important to teach your child to swim. As parents we can enlist the help of behavior therapists to work on safety skills, and we can work on them at home.

As a mom one of the best things I have done for my peace of mind is to make sure David has a tracking device in case he wanders. David's tracker is provided to him by the local police department. Although I am grateful for the donors who make the program possible, I am now looking at GPS tracking devices I can monitor myself from my phone. There are a variety of tracking devices, and parents must decide which GPS will meet the needs of their family best. Below is a list of trackers.[5] Of these I have only tried the Angel Sense GPS, which was great. In addition to tracking, it also offers a voice component, so you can listen in on your child's environment when he or she is not with you. The downside to Angel Sense, and many other trackers, is that they are water resistant, not waterproof. David's first (expensive) Angel Sense tracker got wet, and I had to replace it (I was locked into a contract). The second tracker got wet while we were at Disneyland, so I spent the rest of our vacation on pins and needles. Angel Sense isn't perfect but has many great attributes.

I am thinking of getting David a Gizmo, by Verizon. The Gizmo is a GPS device that will alert you if your child is out of a designated area. For example, your child should be at school from 8:30 a.m. to 3:00 p.m. If they leave the school address, you will be notified. The Gizmo allows for up to four phone contacts and takes incoming calls as well.

There are a number of great products on the market. Determining which one will work best for your family is your call. If cost is an issue, your local disability resource center may be able to help with funding.

GPS tracking devices

hereO GPS Watch
AngelSense
AmbyGear Smartwatch
Weenect Kids GPS
Tinitell
My Buddy Tag
PocketFinder
Lineable
Amber Alert GPS Locator
TraxPlay
KOREX Waterproof Babysitter
GizmoGadget
GIZMOPAL 2
Kigo Watch
dokiWatch

In addition to working with our kids on safety aware-ness and teaching them to swim, there are other things we can do to keep our kids safe. When David was little, he seemed to be on a daily mission to escape from the house. We added two locks to every door, which helped until he fig-ured out he could push a chair over to the door and unlock them himself. I ended up buying cheap door alarms from the Dollar Store (they may also sell them at your local hard-ware store) and putting them on every door that he could exit. The nice thing about the cheap door alarms is that you can take them on vacation and put them on your hotel door. I also used to bring them to family events so I would know if he was trying to escape.

When I bought my house several years back, I had a security system added to my home so I am alerted when a door or window has been opened. Taking these precautions has allowed me to relax in my own home, something that was impossible before door alarms. Wandering can take a tremendous toll on caregivers, and it's important for us to take the necessary steps to ensure we can maintain a sense of peace in our homes and when our children are away from us. If you are concerned about your child while she is at school, a tracker can help, but keep in mind, you can add wandering concerns to their IEP or Behavior Plan as well. Additionally, the National Autism Association has a tool-kit for teachers which includes door alarms, picture cards, etc.[6]

As the years go by, relationships will come and go. We will be stared at in public, and we will learn to handle it gracefully. We will change how we approach holidays and vacations, and we will appreciate the need to maintain our own physical and mental health. As the years go by, you will find that what lies within you is greater than what lies behind you and what lies before you, and it is greater than the bad days you have. What lies within you is the ability to stay positive, to stay focused, and to reclaim your life.

NOTES FOR CHAPTER 8

9

LEGAL CONSIDERATIONS

Injustice anywhere is a threat to justice every-where.

—Dr. Martin Luther King, Jr.

LEARNING THE LAW as it pertains to children with autism is not as daunting as it may seem. Over the years, I have learned disability law incrementally. I didn't tackle it all at once. There are many aspects of the law you will need to know, but you don't need a law degree to grasp the basics. This chapter is a brief rundown of legal documents and statutes you will want to familiarize yourself with. Even a basic understanding of our child's legal rights will help ensure they are protected while we are able to care for them and when we are gone. Our children can be subject to great injustice. Learning the law will help protect their rights and secure their possessions as they enter adulthood.

On your quest to provide your child with the best life possible, you will need to find your tribe. It is in the parent groups and by having conversations with people who have walked in our shoes that we learn the most. Your allies, your mentors, and your real-life heroes will be found in the autism community. It is important to get out and socialize when possible and to make meaningful connections on Facebook or online parent groups. Some of the most valuable connections I have made were from speaking to other parents and attending autism conferences. When I attended the TACA conference for chapter coordinators in October of 2016, I knew I had found my tribe. TACA is made up primarily of volunteers, so every person I met was genuinely concerned about the well-being of people with autism and their families. The conference included speakers from all over the country who addressed a variety of topics. There were classes on diet, genetic mutations, digestive system issues, neurological issues, bullying, RPM, and everything in between.

The most valuable lesson I learned there was about the importance of special needs trusts. As I sat through the class on special needs trusts and guardianship, I felt like I had been slapped with a proverbial dose of reality. Every child with autism, unless they are extremely high functioning, needs to have either a special needs trust established or an ABLE account (a tax-advantaged savings account for the benefit of disabled people). Additionally, guardianship, in the case that you can no longer care for the child, must be established in writing with an attorney.

In addition to legally binding documents such as special needs trusts, there are many other legal considerations parents must be aware of. As an advocate, I often see there are serious legal issues revolving around people with autism and victimization. There are legal matters pertaining to schools, public places, and our children's legal rights under IDEA and the ADA.

You do not need to be a lawyer to understand the law or to defend your child's rights. Once you know the law, you will start to see cracks in the system. In my experience, school principals rarely read the ADA and IDEA and will unknowingly circumvent the law in some instances. Unless a police department makes it a point to train their officers in the ADA, police officers would have no way of knowing that our children have different rights than the average citizen. When you take your child to an amusement park, the sixteen-year-old working the rides probably hasn't read the ADA and, therefore, may be unable to provide your child with reasonable accommodations.

Knowing the ADA, IDEA, and the basics of special needs trusts and guardianship has the potential of changing the course of your child's life. For years, I operated under the assumption that schools, public entities, and police departments were well versed in the ADA. It wasn't until I started doing advocacy work that I realized that people trying to marginalize or prosecute people with autism had *never* read the ADA. As parents we can't assume that the professionals we encounter have a solid background in disability law.

This chapter will give you an overview of disability law and trusts. As time goes on, the links provided in the endnotes will prove to be useful. As legal matters arise, know that there are often inexpensive ways to address these matters. By accessing the sites provided, reaching out to disability law attorneys, reading law books (so fun), and taking courses on the ADA, you will have the advantage of knowing the law better than many of the professionals you encounter.

In order to successfully navigate our way through the maze of disability law, we need to get organized. So, here it is, the list of things parents and guardians need to know for chapter 9:

- The basics of special needs trusts and guardianship
- Making the most of the Americans with Disabilities Act (ADA)
- Addressing victimization and criminal matters

THE BASICS OF SPECIAL NEEDS TRUSTS AND GUARDIANSHIP

Of the many people I met at the TACA conference, one of the people who stood out the most was a man named Marc

Ang. Marc is a financial and estate planner who founded Mangus Finance in California. He was at the conference providing information on estate planning for families affected by autism. I asked him a million questions, and being the wonderful person that he is, he took time out of his day to help me better understand the complexities of estate planning for children with autism. He is in California; if you are local he can help provide you with information pertaining to financial planning. If you are out of state, you can access his website at www.mangusfinance.com. The website offers a life insurance calculator and estate plan preparedness quiz for parents; these tools can help you clarify the type of estate plan you will need and how much money your child will need as an adult.[1]

Marc, like every other person I met at TACA, just wants to help our community and improve the lives of people with autism. His website offers valuable information for parents at no cost and will provide you with enough information to start setting up the framework for your child's estate. When it comes to estate planning, it's important to find someone to work with who is a good, decent human being. These are complex issues and finding the right person to walk you through them is a must. If I were in California, Marc would be my go-to person; he's smart, organized, and caring, just the type of person you need to help guide you through estate planning. Marc and other people who work in his field can help guide you through financial planning and protecting your child's assets, and in the case that you need a trust, an attorney will help you with that process.

There are two primary factors to consider when determining which type of trust your child will need: your child's ability to care for himself and your assets.

If your child is on the high-functioning end of the spectrum and is on the road to independence, a special needs trust or ABLE account may not be necessary.

However, if he or she will be eligible for government benefits, trust planning is needed.

If your child with autism is unable to care for himself and you have few assets, you can focus on guardianship (which I will get to later) and setting up an ABLE account. ABLE accounts were established under the *Achieving a Better Life Experience Act* of 2014. This type of account allows parents or family members to put aside up to $100,000 in an account to be used for the child's care. An ABLE account is not taxed and will not impact SSI benefits as long as the account balance stays under $100,000. You can learn more at, http://www.ablenrc.org/about/what-are-able-accounts.[2]

If your child with autism is unable to care for herself and you have a significant asset base (your assets exceed $100,000)—this applies to any homeowner, even if your equity is low—and your child is considered disabled, you will need a special needs trust for two objectives. First, to avoid having your child's government benefits threatened and, second, to avoid having your assets go to the money pit known as probate court.

As an example, if your home is worth $300,000 and you owe $150,000, the assets that will be counted against your child's SSI will be $300,000. If you put your home (using this example) in a special needs trust, your child can continue to live in the home and the value will not be counted against their SSI and Medicaid (assuming they receive Medicaid benefits).

If your child directly inherits the home and it is not in a trust, Medicaid can count the real property value of $300,000 against the child's Medicaid, triggering a payback. In summary, if your child inherits a home that is not in a trust, he will lose SSI and Medicaid and be expected to reimburse Medicaid.

If you find yourself on the cusp of needing either a special needs trust or ABLE account, it's important to reach out to attorneys in your state and clarify your state's laws pertaining to disability-related trusts and the maximum amount of assets your child can have without triggering probate court (probate court is a specialized type of court which manages the debt and property of the deceased). To figure out where your state's thresholds are, you can refer to this handy list: http://www.mangusfinance.com/probate-state-by-state-thresholds-limits/.

Once you have established whether you need an ABLE account or special needs trust or both (you may want to complete the estate plan preparedness quiz at mangusfinance.com to make this determination), you will want to reach out to an attorney who works specifically with special needs planning and estates. Finding the right attorney for your trust is important. Attorneys, like Elizabeth McCoy in California, focus on special needs trusts and know state laws pertaining to people with disabilities well. Finding an attorney like Elizabeth is key. She attends TACA conferences and is a TACA Board Member. She knows what our kids lives are like and is genuinely concerned for their well-being.

Although none of us wants to think about what will happen to our children when we are gone, it is important to plan for this inevitability. There are very few resources for adults with disabilities, and the little help that is available to them is often not enough to cover the costs of food, clothing, recreation, and other expenses of living. Most of us don't have much money in the bank, but the little we do have and any equity we may have in our home, for example, can be allocated into a trust and used to provide for our children with autism when we no longer can.

Special needs trusts are not cheap to set up; fees range from two to three thousand dollars on average. If you cannot afford to have a trust drawn up, your disability resource center may, on rare occasions, or you can reach out to your local Autism Society, The Arc, or even Parent to Parent for ideas on how to approach this in the least expensive way. It's not always easy for us to come up with the money for these things, but, hey, not much about this journey is easy and yet we persevere. Never give up!

In addition to setting up special needs trusts and protecting our kids financially, we *must* establish guardianship of our children in the event we can no longer care for them. States have some differences in their definitions of guardianship and conservatorship. In most cases a guardian oversees the needs of the person with autism (or other disability) and the conservator oversees all financial matters. However, in some states the conservator is both guardian and financial conservator. Because why make it easy, right?

I will use "guardian" as the person who cares for the child and "conservator" as the person who oversees financial matters. Once you start the process of guardianship and conservatorship, your state's definition of guardian and conservator will be made clear either by the court documents you file or by the attorney who helps you file the legal paperwork involved. You can also Google guardianship in your state and links to applicable legal documents should come up.

It is critical to establish a guardian for your child. It is not expensive and will eliminate the possibility of your child ending up in state-run care, if that is not your wish. Guardianship of a person with autism is dependent on the affected person's ability to make medical and financial decisions for himself. If a person with autism is able to care for themselves and they can get to work, keep up with housework, grocery shop, etc., they do not require a guardian. If, however, a person with autism is a minor or is unable to care for their own needs as an adult, guardianship should be established by the parent or caregiver. The people best able to care for our children are most likely family members and friends. The guardian for our child with autism should be chosen by us and not left to the courts. We know our child best and can determine who would provide the best care. If you do not have family or a friend to assign guardianship to, the courts can assign a public guardian, or a county agency can be named as guardian. Many of us struggle with whom to ask to be our child's guardian. If you do not have family or friends to ask, you might want to consider an aide from school or therapist who you trust. Sometimes these matters require thinking outside the box.[3]

A conservator of the estate, in this example, is a person who oversees financial matters on behalf of the person with autism. The conservator monitors all financial matters and manages all assets. If, however, you establish a special needs trust, the trustee will manage financial matters.[4]

MAKING THE MOST OF THE AMERICANS WITH DISABILITIES ACT

The Americans with Disabilities Act (ADA) gives civil rights protections to people with qualifying disabilities. Autism is a qualifying diagnosis in many cases. David certainly qualifies for protections under the ADA, and many people who have substantial mental or physical impairments that limit major life activities will qualify for protections under the ADA as well.

Most of us think of the ADA in terms of employment. Employers are required by law to make reasonable accommodations for their employees who have a disability. Before I had a child with autism, I always thought of the ADA as providing for physical accommodations for people with physical disabilities such as deafness or paraplegia. However, the ADA applies to multiple disabilities and can serve as a means of keeping our children with autism employed.

For people with autism, a reasonable accommodation might mean that the employer provides, or allows for, noise-blocking headphones during the work day. A reasonable accommodation for a person with autism may include shorter work days or a modified schedule. Many tech companies prefer to hire people with autism and are happy to make accommodations. People with autism tend to do well in the tech industry for a number of reasons: they often have an acute attention to detail, can be very regimented and follow their job description to a T, and they are frequently drama-free and do not contribute to office politics and infighting. In many ways, people with autism can be the perfect employee. Finding the right company, which sees value in their work and who will happily make accommodations is key. There are companies who want to hire our kids; if the first few job applications are denied, don't get discouraged. There is a company out there that needs the skills your kid brings to the table.

In regard to employment, BCBAs, OTs and disability resource centers can collectively help transition a person with autism to a new position and can help with job coaching. Potential employers may be set at ease if we assure them professionals are available to help if our kids are struggling in some capacity. The ADA does not require a company to hire a person with a disability, but it does disallow discrimination in the hiring process and requires employers make reasonable accommodations for people with autism and other qualifying disabilities. Although some companies may be hesitant to hire someone with autism, most are pleasantly surprised at the diligence and fastidiousness of our kids. And as an added benefit, companies may qualify for a tax credit if they hire a person with a qualifying disability under the ADA.[5]

Public entities, including places such as schools, grocery stores, and day care centers, are required to make accommodations as well. Accommodations under the ADA apply only to public entities and do not include private clubs, churches, and other privately funded organizations.

Public accommodations can be hugely beneficial to people with autism. One example is waiting in line. When David was little we stayed locked inside our home until I found out about reasonable accommodations under the ADA. It opened up the world for us; they meant that David could go out and experience the things other kids his age were enjoying. When I first read the ADA, I was thrilled; I knew it would change everything for the better.

For example, here in Colorado there are a million fun things to do around the holidays. We were never able to participate in any of these activities because David was unable to wait in lines. When he was about six, he found a picture of the Denver Zoo Lights, our city zoo's extensive Christmas light display and kept handing it to me. Emboldened with this new ADA information, I called the Denver Zoo and asked to speak to a manager. I explained that my son had autism but was unable to wait in line. Before I could even give a lengthy speech about reasonable accommodations, he said, "We'd love to have your family. Just come to Guest Services and explain that your child has a disability and cannot wait in line." When we got to the Denver Zoo, we went straight to the Guest Services desk. I handed them a letter specifying his disability and helpful accommodations, and guess what? They walked us to the front of the line, and it was no problem.

That was a valuable learning experience for me. I had spent years agonizing over our inability to go out in public and what David was being denied as a child. Knowing just the basics of the ADA allowed me to open up a whole new world for him. Public accommodations are intended to help our kids access public facilities and participate in typical childhood activities.

How we approach reasonable accommodations is important. We can't expect the teenager working at the movie theater to know federal statutes, so it's best to call ahead of time if possible and speak to a manager. If we speak to a manager or business owner before arriving, it can make the process painless. Over the years, I have learned that we catch more bees with honey. People are far more likely to be helpful and accommodating if we are kind and polite. My dad always told me, "Most people never hear anything nice about themselves. When you give a person a compliment, it is no sweat off of your back, but it may change their entire day. Because it's so rare hearing something nice about themselves can be a very powerful motivator, and you will get more cooperation by being kind than you would otherwise." I have always heeded my dad's advice. We all need to hear more nice things about ourselves. People quickly become more cooperative and are more likely to help our children when we build them up. In the link in the endnotes,[6] you will find a very simple yet concrete explanation of your child's rights under the ADA. Again, you don't have to be a lawyer to defend your child's rights; you just need to know the basics.

The Individuals with Disabilities Education Act (IDEA) falls under the umbrella of the ADA. Any reasonable accommodation listed in the ADA applies to schools as well. I wouldn't count on your school's principal or even special ed department having read the ADA or IDEA recently. As an advocate I have been in IEP and disciplinary meetings where I backed the principal into the corner and gave them no choice but to admit they hadn't read IDEA or the ADA in years. It is our responsibility to know the law and make sure public entities are in adherence with the ADA. If you feel that your child's rights have been violated and you are not comfortable addressing this on your own, you can reach out to legal advocates, attorneys, Parent to Parent, The Arc or your local Autism Society chapter for advice.

ADDRESSING VICTIMIZATION AND CRIMINAL MATTERS

While extremely important, the topic of victimization is very difficult for me to address. My worries about people victimizing my son are well founded. My son has been lost by a day care and mistreated at school, and nothing was done about it. If it happened now, I would make sure the people who hurt him were prosecuted to the fullest extent of the law. Unfortunately, the damage is done, and I can't go back and have these people prosecuted. There was a time when he came home from a place (if I say where I will be sued as he cannot testify) covered in handprint bruises. I knew who was doing it, but because David couldn't testify social services did nothing. When he was at day care, I walked into a dramatic scene where one of the day care employees was being fired. She looked at me and yelled, "One of the reasons they are firing me is because I said I was going to tell you what was going on around here! (She-who-is-not-to-be-named) is lazy and has lost your son three times. Last time he was a block away when I found him."

I asked the day care owner what her employee was talking about, and she quickly shut the office door on me. I took David home, and then I fell apart. It was literally the only day care that would take a child who wandered, had life-threatening food allergies, had autism, was violent, and nonverbal. I called every day care remotely near my home or job, and no one would take him. My choice was to stop working and have no money to live and pay for his biomedical interventions or allow him to go somewhere I now realized was unsafe for him. It was a horrible feeling, and I wasn't able to sleep much at all the following week. I finally decided to resign my position and hope to God I could find part-time work while David was in school.

That is our reality. We have to work, but few people or daycare centers are capable of caring for our kids. Then, if we take government assistance, we are called lazy and told we are "milking the system." Sometimes it's going to feel like every option is a crappy one. However, when we are forced to come up with creative solutions to work and find childcare, it can be done. It takes time and creative thinking, but there is always a way to make things work.

Victimization is a serious problem in our community. Our kids don't make very good witnesses, nor can they provide police with detailed accounts of events if they have been victimized. According to VERA Institute of Justice, people with disabilities are more likely to be victims of crime for the following reasons:

> *They appear to be easy targets, unable to protect themselves.*
> *They are taught compliance from an early age.*
> *Many people with disabilities—especially people who have intellectual or cognitive disabilities— are taught to follow the directions of others, usually with the intent of ensuring that they cope effectively with daily life and for their safety.*
> *This conditioning, however, may also increase their vulnerability to abuse.*
> *Concern about retaliation by caregivers or about losing caregivers/family members.*
> *Concern that they will be institutionalized.*
> *Concern that they will be referred to Adult Protective Services.*[7]

The reality is that about thirty percent of people with autism who interact with police departments are nonverbal. This makes it difficult for police officers to file criminal charges against a possible perpetrator. Additionally, people with disabilities who can speak fear reporting victimization for the following reasons:

Their voices are often silenced.
They may not have channels to report their victimization on their own.
Despite suffering and negative outcomes, they may not label what's happening as victimization.
They may depend on perpetrators for survival, care, and housing.
Their rates of victimization are often very high.
Their access to informed help sources is often very limited.[8]

Because victimization in our communities is prevalent, it's important to take steps to protect our children. As a mother and advocate for people with autism, I can say with certainty that the most important thing you can do for your child is teach her to communicate. The phonics song I shared can help build a language base for intensive speech therapy. Some children who may never speak can learn the alphabet and therefore learn to spell. They need some way to communicate to their caregivers if they feel unsafe or have been harmed by another person.

Additionally, there are tracking devices that can also serve as a speaker of sorts. Some GPS trackers come with sound options, so you can listen in on your child's environment. If you are concerned about your child's well-being in certain settings, having the option to listen in on their surroundings may help give you some clarity as to what is occurring throughout their day.

The Arc has resources for families on how to avoid victimization. They also have helpful materials available online at no cost. The Arc explains that the best way to keep our kids safe is to help avoid victimization in the first place. They recommend that the people who work with our children have access to information pertaining to victims' rights. They go on to say:

> Cross-training needs to occur among all profes-
> sionals in schools, police departments, victim
> assistance agencies and in the courtroom as
> a way to start opening the lines of communica-
> tion between these systems. Consider contacting
> your school's special education department and
> request that this training be offered if it is cur-
> rently unavailable.[9]

The reality is, most agencies who work with our children are not trained to identify signs of victimization, nor
are they prepared to address it legally.

Some Arc chapters provide training on criminal justice
issues to a variety of agencies. If you are interested in your
child's school or local police department having access to
training materials or receiving training, reach out to an Arc
chapter in your state or contact the national Arc for more
information. If you would like to read the information for
yourself and pass it along to local agencies, you can access
it in the link in the endnotes.[10]

As parents we want to protect our children. Sometimes as parents of children with autism, this means reaching out to our local police department or child's school.
Schools and police departments are not always well versed
in addressing victimization of people with autism. The
more information they have, the better they can address
this issue.

In terms of criminal matters, the justice system is a
hot mess as it pertains to people with autism. Because our
kids often have no physical symptoms of a disability, they
are given no opportunity to speak to a disability advocate
or attorney. They are often convicted of crimes they did
not commit or confess to things they did not do. They are

taught to be compliant, and in an effort to comply and make people happy, they may comply with whatever they think is being asked of them.

The justice system is not set up to benefit or account for people with autism. High-functioning people with autism appear to be cognitively aware of their actions and are perceived to be capable of criminal conduct. I find that is generally not the case. In over ten years of working with families affected by autism and having worked one-on-one with hundreds of families, I have never met a person with autism who has an ounce of malice inside them. Furthermore, I have never met one person with autism who is capable of knowingly committing a crime. Are they talked into doing bad things? Yes. Do their peers talk them into doing bad things for entertainment? Yes. Have most of the kids I work with been told what crime is? No. They are supremely innocent and should be protected by the criminal justice system, not prosecuted by it. That's not to say that there are no people with autism who may intentionally commit crimes. However, in my ten years of working with people on the spectrum, I have yet to meet one person with autism I felt was capable of knowingly committing a crime, competent to stand trial, or could adhere to the parameters of probation. They need protection, not prosecution.

When a person with autism is questioned by police, things can go really badly, really fast. People with autism usually want to comply and make the police officer happy, so they tell them whatever they think the officer wants to hear. According to The Arc:

> As suspects, individuals with this disability are frequently used by other criminals to assist in lawbreaking activities without understanding their involvement in a crime or the consequences of their involvement. They may also have a strong need to be accepted and may agree to help with criminal

activities in order to gain friendship. Many individuals unintentionally give misunderstood responses to officers, which increase their vulnerability to arrest, incarceration and possibly execution, even if they committed no crime (Perske, 2003).[11]

It's also important to know our child's rights in case they are ever detained and/or charged with a crime. There are certain procedures that must be adhered to, but again, unless a police department has read the ADA as it pertains to people with disabilities, they may not know the differences in our children's legal rights and the legal rights of the general population. In The Arc's *Criminal Justice Advocacy Booklet*, they explain:

Police officers and court officials often do not realize that a majority of those affected by intellectual disabilities are mildly affected (approximately 88%) and will not readily appear as having a disability. For that reason, a number of "checklists" have been created to help officers identify the presence of a disability.

For example, an officer can find out if the person:

Refers to a caseworker/staff/friend at a center or group home;
Receives SSI;
Has an ID that provides a phone number to call;
Appears too open to being led by others or too eager to agree or please the questioning Officer;
Has difficulty communicating events in his or her own words (without parroting or mimicking responses);
Seems overly awed or intimidated by the police uniform, badge, gun, etc.; or
Seems to agree to everything asked of him or her.[12]

265

There are ways in which police officers can identify whether or not a person has a developmental disability, including autism. Once a person with autism is convicted, they often violate their probation. They may be unable to drive themselves to required meetings or to even keep up with the required paperwork and documents. If incarcerated, they tend to do longer sentences because without proper support they are unable to keep up with the demands placed on them. I have worked with police departments regarding autism and related wandering issues. In my experience, police officers are invested in our community and genuinely want to do what is best for our kids. When it comes to your local police department, maybe the best thing you can do is bake some cookies, bring them a copy of the *Criminal Justice Advocacy Booklet* and ask if you can volunteer or do anything to help increase autism awareness in your city.

Often, there is no one advocating for our kids. In those times that person may have to be you. Is it intimidating for me to walk into a police station, a senator's office, or legislative hearing? Yes, it is. Being brave and doing the right thing doesn't mean you won't be intimidated or afraid. Bravery means doing what needs to be done in spite of fear. The person who will need to educate police officers in your community might just be you. Know that police are more receptive to helping our kids than you may think, and your help and volunteer hours will be appreciated. (On a side note, I think volunteer work is best done when our kids are getting well and it is not a burden to us.)

If your child does get arrested, he needs to have an advocate with him at the police station. The Arc states:

> The most critical thing to remember during this stage is to make sure individuals with the disabilities have a support person who is familiar with them and their disability to help before and during this stage. So often, suspects with developmental disabilities

have no advocates (or they get one too late after an investigation has begun) and therefore miscommunications or other misunderstandings leave them without a fair and adequate way of defending themselves. Advocates should have a basic understanding of the criminal justice process or find someone who can help navigate them through the process effectively.[13]

If your child with autism is arrested or detained, it is important that she have an advocate or support person present during questioning. She may confess to something she didn't do, or her language and social skills deficits can be misinterpreted as noncompliance. If a person with autism is arrested, they may not understand Miranda Rights and will need to have an advocate or attorney present to check for understanding. If you have a disability law center in your state or county, reach out to them and explain that you need an attorney present while your child is being read her Miranda Rights.

If a person with autism is charged with a crime and is expected to stand before a judge, it's important to know your state's laws as they pertain to competency for standing trial or entering a plea. If set for incarceration, a good attorney or advocate will ask the court to provide an alternative placement to jail or prison if one is available. They can ask that your child be placed in a medical unit or in protective custody.[14]

The large majority of people with autism should not be charged with crimes. The fact is that they are often charged and convicted of crimes after having no accommodations made for them as required by the ADA. That is the antithesis of justice. The purpose of law is to, in laymen's terms, "get the bad guys." In my experience, most people with autism are not capable of being "the bad guy." Yes, there may be that .00001% of people with autism who are capable of intentionally committing a crime, but most are not.

THE AUTISM HELP BOOK

As Martin Luther King Jr. said, "Injustice anywhere is a threat to justice everywhere." People who are incapable of *mens rea* and lack criminal intent should not be charged and convicted of crimes they literally are unable to comprehend. That is an injustice.

How will this change? Who will change it? Perhaps that person is you. Maybe it is you who needs to reach out to your state senator or representative and ask him or her to sponsor a bill that requires police departments and judges to be educated in the ADA as it pertains to people with autism. Maybe it's you who needs to educate your child's school or your local police department. We all go through phases. If you are going through a phase where you are worn out and tired, now is not the time for community outreach. If, however, you are in an ambitious, energetic phase, get out there and change the world. It's waiting for you.

Whether we are setting up a special needs trust or addressing legal matters on behalf of our child with autism, the objective is the same: we want what is just and right for our child. Taking steps to protect your child through trusts and guardianship is critical to his future well-being as an adult. Advocating for our child's legal rights may not be something we planned for, but it is something we can prepare for by learning the ADA and reaching out to local disability organizations.

"Injustice anywhere is a threat to justice everywhere." In our efforts to be the best parents possible, we can take steps to ensure our children have the justice they deserve in this world. We can protect them by choosing the right guardians and putting their assets in a trust. We can protect them by making sure our local police departments, schools, and courts have access to and knowledge of the ADA. We can help protect them with disability advocates and attorneys. Justice for our kids requires diligence, persistence, and the one thing they need the most, someone who loves them enough to go out and change the world for them. That someone is you.

NOTES FOR CHAPTER 9

10

LIFE WITH AUTISM

I've listened enough. It's time for me to speak, however it may sound. Through an electronic device, my hands, or my mouth. Now it's your time to listen. Are you ready?

—Neal Katz, self-advocate

DAVID HAS GONE FROM being severely impacted by autism to now being high-functioning. Once our kids feel well enough to communicate, we can get a chance to know them for the beautiful, complex, and angelic people they really are.

Up to this point this book has been about helping you to understand and organize the many logistical aspects of having a child with autism. The intention of this chapter, however, is to give you a glimpse into the world of autism.

Until I read *Thinking in Pictures* by Temple Grandin, I didn't fully grasp how much my son was absorbing. We don't often get the opportunity to know how people with autism think or what they feel.

I have given you a roadmap to guide you through the complexities of services, therapies, diet, insurance, law, and puberty. I hope that what I have shared with you can help you, in some small way, to allow yourself the grace to feel peace and calm again. This chapter is last because you, as a parent, need to be grounded in order to take this information in, process it, and use it to better understand and connect with your child. You may have noticed that throughout the book I have never referred to either your child or mine, as "being autistic." Autism is just a word for a set of behaviors and commonly outward displays of under-lying medical conditions. Autism is just a word; it does not define or begin to encompass the brilliant, sensitive, kind, and loving person who lies beneath the perceptions of what it is to have autism.

As parents, it is up to us to find ways to be our child's best friend, confidant, and interpreter. For those of us who have semi-verbal children, much of what we know about our child may have been deduced from a series of behaviors, four-word sentences, gestures, and prompted speech. Fil-tering through their complex forms of communication can be difficult but necessary. My hope is that this chapter can help you connect with your child and enable you to identify her emotions when she cannot express how she feels.

Here's what we'll cover about life with autism from the perspective of a person with autism:

- Understanding the effects of sensory stimuli
- Emotions and autism
- Communication

UNDERSTANDING THE EFFECTS OF SENSORY STIMULI

Unless we are in an extraordinarily loud and chaotic environment, sensory stimuli are no big deal for us. For a person with autism, sensory stimuli can be debilitating and painful. Timothy Ryan is a young man with autism who uses Rapid Prompt Movement (RPM) to communicate. This is a journal entry about his trip to Disneyland which I found to be very helpful in understanding David's perspective on sensory stimuli:

The Disney Park was hot, steamy, muggy, and smelly. My family and I were waiting for the Splash Mountain ride. I felt sick. My body was on fire from the inside out. My head was going to explode. I couldn't talk and describe the agony. That was only the beginning of my ordeal. The airplane would prove to be my greatest challenge thus far. Little did I know everything would go askew.

The airplane was cramped, dirty, noisy, and uncomfortable. Cigarette smoke lingered in the cabin. I became sick, nauseous, and disoriented. Passengers were staring at me with ugly faces. It felt like I was on display at the museum. Dad was aware of my discomfort due to relentless pummeling from my fists. Mom was mortified by my seemingly irrational behavior. My brother Mark slinked down in his seat not saying a word. The flight attendant roamed up and down the aisles glaring in my direction, her arms on her hips with eyes bugging out.

I felt as if my body was breaking down like an old used car. It hurt to breathe, think, talk, and be around people. People make it impossible for me to interact. They speak too rapidly and don't wait for me to respond. If only they would notice how I am trying to fit in and be more typical. It would help if people made an effort to get to know me. I am suffering from an illness that robs me from establishing relationships. I can feel rejection. It hurts to see others move forward while I remain trapped in my inner world. It is not my choice to be disabled and dependent upon people.[1]

Here we have a perfect example of what we could easily perceive to be negative behavior. No one with autism is intentionally trying to ruin your day. They are often in pain and unable to convey their feelings of frustration and unrest. Sensory stimuli can be painful for people with autism. Timothy describes the sensory stimulation at Disneyland as agonizingly painful. It is clear that he is acutely aware of those around him. He makes clear his psyche is impacted by the stares of others, "Passengers were staring at me with ugly faces. It felt like I was on display at the museum...I can feel rejection."

Timothy's account of his trip to Disneyland is hard to read but something we all need to be aware of. If our kids are seen as "misbehaving" (whether they are our minor or adult children), it's important to take a step back and assess the sensory stimuli they have been exposed to. Say you just left a busy shopping mall and your child is "misbehaving." Now try to imagine their behavior in terms of how agonizingly painful sensory stimuli may have affected them.

Temple Grandin explains her experience with auditory processing like this:

> *My hearing is like having a hearing aid with the volume control stuck on "super loud." It is like an open microphone that picks up everything. I have two choices: turn the mike on and get deluged with sound or shut it off.*[2]

Temple's experience with sound is similar to the experiences of many people with autism. One young man told me he heard every sound at the same decibel level. He said the noise of a fan, the traffic outside, the TV in another room and the sound of people talking all came in at the same decibel level. Every person with autism is different, and their experiences with sensory input are different as well. Often what we perceive to be negative behavior is simply their response to being overstimulated. Noise-blocking headphones can help decrease some of the auditory stimulation if necessary.

Temple goes on to describe her tactile experiences as well:

> As a child in church, skirts and stockings drove me crazy. My legs hurt during the cold winter when I wore a skirt. The problem was the change from pants all week to a skirt on Sunday. If I had worn skirts all the time, I would not have been able to tolerate pants. Today I buy clothes that feel similar. My parents had no idea why I behaved so badly. A few simple changes in clothes would have improved my behavior.[3]

And there it is. A few simple changes in her clothes could have prevented the negative behavior. As parents, we are often guessing at why our child is misbehaving, screaming, throwing themselves down, or kicking our butts in some other fashion. As our kids' health improves and their communication abilities improve, we can get a glimpse into their world. Their day-to-day life is often literally painful. The best we can do to help them with sensory processing issues is to go through a process of elimination and/or keep a written journal of behaviors. If your child screams every time you put a pair of jeans on him, try sweat pants. If they rip the tags off of shirts, buy tag less shirts. Eliminate possible sensory triggers wherever possible.

Keeping a journal can be a powerful and useful tool to help you understand your child. Journals allow us to see patterns we might otherwise miss in our day-to-day lives. Keeping a journal on behavior and sensory triggers does not have to be formal or complicated. For a couple of years, I tracked David's behavior in a spiral notebook I bought for fifty cents. I would write down (when possible) his behavior and what happened prior to the behavior. Through the log,

I discovered that he melted down every time I took him to Costco, my local grocery store, or the health food store up the street. One day, it occurred to me that all three places used fluorescent lighting. I stopped taking him to those stores until we were a year into detox. When we tried again, he did much better with the negative effects of fluorescent lighting.

It is imperative that we are mindful of sensory stimuli and the environments we take our children into. Yes, it can limit our social lives, but socializing will come in time. Once they start to heal, getting out in public becomes a bit easier. Occupational therapy and the Wilbargar Brushing Technique can help but will take time. It's possible your child's sensory processing difficulties may never disappear entirely but can be greatly decreased.

A great example of sensory overload is found in a video by Carly Fleischman, mentioned in chapter 3. In the video, she demonstrates what it is like to feel overstimulated in a public place. Another video providing a glimpse into what it's like to live with sensory processing deficits was made by a young boy named Alexander Marshall. This video is only about a minute and a half long, and it's difficult to watch it to the end. At the end of the video the boy proclaims, "I am not naughty, I am autistic, and I just get too much information." The links to both videos can be found in the endnotes.[4]

Our kids are not naughty. They are not misbehaving. They are struggling. The most notable part of Alexander Marshall's video for me was the image of the boy counting on his fingers. I interpreted the counting as a "stim" (self-stimulatory behavior). For all the years David stimmed, I rarely tried to stop him as I knew his stimming was his way of coping with his environment. If our kids flap their hands, jump, clap, etc., it has a function for them that can enable them to control, on some level, their response to being overstimulated.

Sensory processing for people with autism is very different from sensory processing for the rest of us. One young man described auditory processing as "stacking." He told me, "Don't ask so many questions. They are stacking up, and I am still trying to answer your first question." When we ask people with autism a question and they don't immediately answer, they may be processing what we said and formulating a response. Processing times vary among our kids; if a child's processing time is fifteen seconds, it will take fifteen seconds to process our question and respond. In that case, repeating the same question will only prolong the response. Like everything else with our kids, there is no simple, easy answer to how we help them through this process. What can be easy is showing them love, compassion, and patience. We must always keep in mind that their brain simply works differently than ours. They don't need us to fix everything. They just need us to love them as they are—stims and all.

I will leave you with a quote on sensory processing from Jenny McCarthy's book *Louder than Words*. When her son was in recovery from autism and started to speak, she asked him why he flapped has hands. He replied, "Because I get so excited and then I fly just like the angels do."[5] Stimming is purposeful and serves a function for our kids. Whether it helps them calm down or fly like the angels do, it has significant meaning to them.

EMOTIONS AND AUTISM

When David was little I sometimes wondered if he felt things the way he did before he regressed. Before he regressed, he interacted with us. He became extremely excited when his dad came home from work. He responded to us by smiling, waiving, and saying "hi" and "bye-bye." After his regression, he no longer seemed interested in us;

he stopped noticing when his dad came in the door and would no longer allow me to hug or touch him (he didn't love hugs before the regression, but after he did not want to be touched in any way).

Because he seemed so detached from his family, I sometimes wondered if he felt emotions the way he'd felt them before the regression. It wasn't until I read, "Beatitudes for Friends of Disabled Children" that I stopped thinking he was free from the emotions he felt before his health was compromised. As parents of children with autism, doctors, relatives, and everyone in between wants to give us advice and make declarations about our kids. One doctor told me to put David in a home because he would "never speak, read, write, or live on his own. He won't even notice you've gone."

What people don't know about autism is shocking, but the things they actually say out of ignorance can be immensely hurtful. No matter what anyone told me or how many doctors swore he was not taking in information, I always remembered how David was before he regressed. I knew that the thinking, feeling, sweet boy was still in there. No dismal prognosis, dismissive doctor, or negative Nancy was going to make me feel any differently.

Years later, when his language was increasing, he looked at me one day and said, "You are the best mother and love me times one million." Had I listened to that doctor, my son would now be in an institution, his emotions and voice locked away for the rest of his life. Sometimes trusting our gut and believing in our child is more powerful than any assertion a professional makes about them. Your child is in there—feeling, thinking, and desperate for understanding. In this instance the doctors were wrong. David was right, I love him "times one million" and never considered putting him in a home or giving up. I knew he was in there, waiting for me to get him out.

Many of our children cannot tell us how they feel; we are left guessing at their emotional state of well-being. The rare glimpse we get of their feelings can be found in the writings of people with autism.

In his book, *The Reason I Jump*, thirteen-year-old Naoki Higashida says:

On our own we simply don't know how to get things done the same way you do things. But, like everyone else, we want to do the best we possibly can. When we sense you've given up on us, it makes us feel miserable. So please keep helping us, through to the end.

...But I ask you, those of you who are with us all day, not to stress yourselves out because of us. When you do this, it feels as if you're denying any value at all that our lives may have—and that saps the spirit we need to soldier on. The hardest ordeal for us is the idea that we are causing grief for other people. We can put up with our own hardships okay, but the thought that our lives are the source of other people's unhappiness, that's plain unbearable.[6]

Because David rarely tells me how he feels, I have had to rely on the accounts of other teenagers with autism for insight into my son's world. Reading *The Reason I Jump* was enormously helpful for me because for the first time I was able to understand how David feels when I stress out over his health, his education, and his future. Since reading Naoki's book, I have stopped talking about his education and the cost of biomedical interventions in front of him. Hearing a young man with autism use the words "miserable," "unhappy," or "unbearable" illuminates just how powerful our words can be. What we say in front of our kids impacts them and their emotional state. Although they may not demonstrate that they understand what we are saying, they frequently do, and they are taking our words to heart.

Another great perspective is from eighteen-year old Tyler McNamer. Tyler wrote *Population One: Autism, Adversity, and the Will to Succeed* in which he offers a unique perspective and gives us the opportunity to learn more about the emotions our children struggle to relay:

> While writing the book, I often felt depressed about a lot of stuff. The way I see it is when thinking about the past and I know I can't relive them, it's really hard. Especially when writing a chapter about my parents divorce it was challenging and I was really sad while writing about those kinds of topics.

He goes on to say:

> I have to remember all the stuff that's going to be in the book like, for example, when I was 3 months old I remembered an iceberg on the Atlantic Ocean while going to Sweden to see my relatives."[7]

Tyler writes about his parents' divorce and shockingly states that he remembers being three months old and going on vacation. Every person with autism is different, but Tyler and my own son seem to have many similar traits and circumstances. David was heartbroken over my divorce. He carried a laminated picture of him and his father everywhere for months. One time, we were in a store and he saw a man who looked like his dad. He ran after him and hugged his leg, refusing to let go. The man looked confused and a little irritated. Tears streaming down my face, I explained that my ex-husband had left and hadn't seen our son in over a year. I told the man he looked strikingly similar to my ex and that my son just missed his dad. Luckily, we were by the toy aisle and I was close enough to run over and grab a toy to distract David. I was able to pry him off the man's leg with the promise of a new toy. We ran to the checkout, David desperately searching around for the man he thought was his father. He screamed all the way to the car and the entire ride home. The answer to the question *Is my son feeling emotions?* was answered that day. Not only did he feel the loss of his dad, but he was actively looking for him while we were in public places.

The point is when we as parents struggle financially or get divorced, our kids are often pushed to the side while we struggle to cope. Knowing the perspective of people with autism has been eye-opening for me. Without that glimpse of what my son may be experiencing I was left grasping at straws about how David felt. Like Tyler, David remembers everything. I know now that he remembers the divorce and everything in between. He is acutely aware of and holds the memory of everything that has happened to him and around him. Deep healing is needed on many levels.

If you have a child who does not speak or express feelings, it is easy to overlook their emotional needs when there is a crisis. A typical child will tell you how they feel. They will cry, ask questions, and hopefully explain ways in which we can help them cope. People with autism, whether they are verbal or not, will have a hard time expressing their emotions in most cases. For example, when David was in first grade and mostly nonverbal, I bought him Thomas the Train tennis shoes. He loved Thomas with a passion, and the shoes were on sale for five dollars. I bought the shoes and thought nothing of it until I went to school with him for lunch. The little boys sitting at his lunch table were pointing and laughing at his shoes. I saw his little heart break. Although he couldn't tell me it bothered him, I knew it did.

After school, I got him in the car and told him we were going to buy him new shoes. On our way into the store, he took his Thomas shoes off and threw them in the trash. I knew at that moment that despite his inability to communicate or express how he felt, he was deeply impacted by the words of his peers.

On another day I was observing at David's school during recess and overheard a group of kids making fun of a child with autism. The child with autism was sent to school in sweat pants that were too small and was wearing a shirt with stains on it (this is not a case of the parents not having money, his parents always dressed nicely and drove brand-new cars). The kids who were making fun of the child with autism were in the wrong, but the child with autism's parents could have taken steps to ensure their child was properly groomed and presentable.

Taking steps to ensure our children are not made to feel less than their peers by keeping up with haircuts (if they will allow it), making sure they are clean when they go to school, brushing their teeth and making sure they have clean clothes that fit can go a long way. When our kids can't tell us if they are being made fun of at school, it is important that we do all we can to boost their self-esteem and make sure they are presentable when we send them to school.

Over the years I have noticed that some parents of children with autism don't have birthday parties for their kids. They may have a small party at home with family, which is fine, but every now and then I feel it's important to save up and have a big, fun party for them. If you don't know enough people to fill a party, make reservations at a hotel, or go to an amusement park. Whatever we have to do to make them feel special and important is critical to their emotional well-being. Going out of our way to make them feel like a king or queen will impact their sense of self-worth for years to come.

COMMUNICATION

With regard to autism and communication, the best way I can describe it is with an analogy. Let's say you wake up with a splitting headache. Sound and touch are painful to you. Your stomach hurts. You can neither speak nor write. You feel awful. Imagine now your ranging emotions.

With no clear way to communicate, how would you tell others how you felt? Would you bang your head to let others know you had a headache? Would you shrink away every time someone tried to hug you, knowing that hug would be painful? Would you stay in a noisy room if the sound of the TV and your family talking was as irritating as nails on a chalkboard? Would you want to eat if your stomach hurt all day?

Sometimes, the best way to know how our kids feel is to try to put ourselves in their shoes. If we can't come up with a simple answer to how we'd communicate without speech or ability to write, how can a child figure that out? The answer is that they can't. Many of the negative behaviors we see in our kids are directly attributable to their inability to communicate. Wouldn't you be angry, throw things, and act out if you were in constant pain and couldn't speak? How must they feel living for years in agonizing silence?

Carly Fleischman does a great job of explaining to us as parents what life with autism is like. She writes, "You don't know what it feels like to be me, when you can't sit still because your legs feel like they are on fire, or it feels like a hundred ants are crawling up your arms." She also says, "People look at me and assume I am dumb because I can't talk."[8]

Communication is necessary to the emotional well-being of our children. Carly gained the skills needed to communicate because her parents were diligent with a rigorous therapy schedule. Having the ability to type opened up her world and allowed her parents to get a glimpse into her world: her life, her emotions, and her sense of being.

It's telling that the way Carly's parents found out she could communicate was her running to a keyboard and typing "hurt" and "help." She had lived in silence for eleven years, and the first direct communication she had with her parents was typing the words "hurt" and "help." How many of our kids would tell us they are in pain or ask for help if they could? I am guessing most of them would say the exact same words. Carly's father's response to the revelation that his child could communicate was, "We were also horrified because for years we had spoken in front of her as if she wasn't there." This father was brave enough to tell the truth. Many parents speak in front of their child with autism as if the child doesn't understand. This is probably one of the worst and most damaging things we can do.[9]

Honoring our children as people and being respectful of their feelings will go a long way in building their sense of self-worth.

Naoki describes it better than I ever could:

The conclusion is that both emotional poverty and an aversion to company are not *symptoms* of autism but *consequences* of autism, its harsh lockdown on self-expression and society's near-pristine ignorance about what's happening inside autistic heads.[10]

Our kids are not incapable of hearing or taking in information, they simply can't always get their words out. They do not want to be isolated; autism isolates them from the people they love. It is truly a devastating disorder in this regard.

The bright side is that if Carly and my son can communicate on some level, most people with autism can too. It requires therapy, patience, and often, biomedical interventions. Communication can open up doors for our kids. A lack of communication can leave them isolated within their own minds. Communication, whether it be through word cards, an app, typing, sign language, or speech will allow your child to express himself and will allow you to get to know your child a little better. Everyone wins.

For most of us, the most desperate desire of our hearts is to hear our child speak. Although David doesn't speak as much as I'd like him to, his speech is enough to allow him to communicate needs, wants and perhaps most importantly, tell me he loves me. David's behaviors decreased before he could communicate and disappeared, for the most part, once he was able to communicate using word cards. Though often a difficult process, you will find creating and building upon communication skills with your child is vitally important.

People with autism are complex and beautiful people. Their sensory processing issues hinder their ability to socialize and interact with the world around them and sometimes thinking outside the box is necessary. I attended an essential oils class for autism, and the speaker mentioned having used tea tree oil, also known as melaleuca, which increased her son's verbal abilities. I recently started using it on David, and it's helping him with language in a very significant way.

In the midst of caring for our children's many physical needs, it's not uncommon for us to overlook their emotional needs. The purpose of this chapter is to help you become aware that our children feel the exact same emotions we do. As you move forward, be continuously mindful of their feelings. Although communication may be slow or seemingly nonexistent, they need us. Your child loves you and may want desperately to talk to you. Facilitating communication and working on these skills will open up doors and change the course of their lives.

All of us are doing the best we can with what we have. There are no simple answers to many of the questions we have as parents, but one thing remains fundamentally true: All children need love, time, and dedication. With a little time, patience, and a whole lot of love, your child can blossom. The dreams you had for your child and for your family may look a little different than you anticipated, but those dreams and your life can be restored. Never give up!

NOTES FOR CHAPTER 10

IN CLOSING

*What lies behind us and what lies before us are
small matters compared to what lies within us.*

—Henry David Thoreau

MY DEAR FRIEND Phil Silberman has been with me through
the journey of writing this book. He has read every word
and is quite familiar with my story. One day while discuss-
ing the book, he looked at me and said, "I am astounded
by you. It's amazing that after all you've been through you
still have a sparkle in your eye and a smile on your face." I
laughed it off and told him that my faith in God has kept me
grounded and hopeful.

The truth is that, as parents of children with autism,
we have to find a way to keep that sparkle in our eye and a
smile on our face. My mom once said, "A mother is as happy
as her sickest child." Until David went through chelation
and dietary changes, I rarely smiled or laughed. Because he
was suffering, I was suffering, and I almost felt guilty being
happy. Although many parents see biomedical interventions as another stressor, these interventions can decrease
autism-related symptoms and, therefore, decrease the
stress we face. Now that David is doing well and the behaviors have disappeared, my sense of peace and calm has
returned.

Recently, however, David had a regression and was
very unhappy. Between him hating his new school and his

recurring parasite issues, he started to lose language and was clearly miserable. I spent a week feeling grumpy and stressed asking myself, *How could this happen? We were so close to recovery!* I decided to take to Facebook and ask for help from my friends who have recovered their kids.

TACA moms and my new warrior friends came out in full force to support me. They reminded me that, although I felt I had done *everything* I could for him, I hadn't. They encouraged me to test for mitochondrial dysfunction and Lyme and to reach out to specialists. Heeding their advice, we are back to running tests and seeing specialists to isolate the cause of his regression. When I thought I had done everything, they reminded me there is more I can do to heal him. One of my TACA moms sent me a meme that read, "You didn't come this far to only come this far." And she was right. I have come too far to turn back now. Recovery is within reach and letting a bump in the road stop us would be an insult to David and to the hard work I have put into his health thus far.

The difference between how I cope with stress now and how I dealt with it initially is vast. In the beginning I was unsure of myself and often felt overwhelmed by the pressure of raising a child with autism. Now, however, when I start to get anxious about David's health, I remember that I have the support of my tribe. Many of my TACA mom friends have recovered their kids and can walk me through the interventions I have not yet tried. I also have Facebook friends who have backgrounds in biology, nutrition, holistic health, allopathic medicine, therapies, and the like. I have the support of parents I have met over the years at autism conferences, picnics and legislative hearings. It has taken several years, but I now feel that I have a support system and people to turn to when we I start to feel apprehensive about the road ahead.

In addition to having support from my tribe, I have gained confidence in myself. Knowing I can make it through a divorce, severe autism, bankruptcy, and healing the child I was told to institutionalize gives me a sense of peace. I know I can figure out whatever comes our way. Experience gives us a newly defined sense of strength and purpose. As time goes on and you find your tribe, you will find that the autism community and other parents are your greatest asset.

Finding like-minded people may not happen overnight, but it will happen. Attending autism-related conferences and community outings will enable you to meet people and find resources. For those of you unable to get out and socialize often, Facebook is a great resource; you can follow TACA, Parent to Parent, The Arc, or any organization you choose to keep you up-to-date with the latest research and events. As the years go by, you will meet people who light your path and you will have the benefit of experience. With experience, you will gain confidence in yourself and your ability to face life's challenges.

With experience I have learned to have faith in myself and in David. Experience has taught me to appreciate David and his incredible resilience. David has been through more than any child should, and yet he is kind and nice. While I may be the backbone of my family, David sets the example by which we all live. His humility and forgiving heart keep the rest of us grounded. If he can endure what he has and remain positive and loving, so can we. Although his recent regression was hard on us all, I have faith that I can resolve whatever medical issues he faces, and I have faith in his ability to weather any storm with dignity and a kind heart.

Although my wish is to end this book with "David has recovered," unfortunately that is not the case. I will end it by telling you that we are okay. I am stronger than I thought I could ever be, David has made tremendous gains since the diagnosis, Aidan is a wonderful brother and the ray of sunshine I needed in my life, and Brooks keeps us on our toes and in search of new adventures. Everything is working out just fine.

When it's all said and done, I am okay. David is okay. You and your child will be okay. You will have days when you feel like you can't make it. You can. You will have days that make you want to curl up in a ball and cry your eyes out. Cry. You will have days when you feel like the bravest, strongest warrior on Earth. You are. You will have days when the goals you set for your child are accomplished. Enjoy it.

You will have good days and bad days. How you cope with the bad days is up to you, but I will leave you with this thought: It is impossible to feel bad and think good thoughts. When you start to feel overwhelmed, be mindful of your thinking. I mean, hey, I have been on the road to recovery with David for eleven years. I watched most of my friends' kids recover, and yet I am still waiting for David to fully recover. How is it that I still have hope after all this time? I have hope because I think positively and remain focused on what I *can* do for him, not what I can't do. I focus on the gains he has made and quickly shift my thoughts when I start to feel down.

Faith in God has kept me grounded more than anything. I have spent countless sleepless nights worrying about people with autism and their families. I pray every day for our babies and for us. In prayer I realized that there are too many people out there suffering for me to *not* write this book. Is writing a book as a single mother of three easy? Heck no. It's one of the hardest things I have ever done. However, my conscience, my heart, and my loyalty to God would not allow me to abandon this project, no matter how many times I wanted to. Christians, true Christians, do not live for themselves; they live to honor God. As a Christian, it is my duty to honor and to serve God's people. The Bible says, "If anyone with earthly possessions sees his brother in need but withholds his compassion from him, how can the love of God abide in him?" I do not have earthly possessions to share with you, but I do have information that can improve your life and the life of your child. I see the needs in our community and, in the spirit of compassion, cannot turn away from those needs.

Although my faith in general has inspired me to write this book, there is one Bible verse in particular that plays over and over in my head: "The King will reply, 'Truly I tell you, whatever you did for one of the least of these brothers and sisters of mine, you did for me.'" (Matthew 25:40; NIV). Another translation is, "What you did to the least of my brethren, you did to Me." Both translations run through my mind on a regular basis. What is done to the least of us, those who are defenseless and unable to care for themselves, is done to God. I cannot, in good conscience, turn from people who are unable to care for themselves. If God has favorites, it's probably people with autism and other disabilities. They are pure at heart, honest, loving, and more like God than I ever will be. They are certainly his beloved, and it is an honor to help ease the burden on them and their parents.

It is through faith that I believed my son could heal, and he has. It is through faith that I know he will recover some day. It is through faith that I wrote this book in hopes that it would reach those who need it most.

When all is said and done, I wrote this book for you. I know that I cannot reach millions of families affected by autism speaking to one parent at a time, so I did the next best thing: I put everything I know into one, hopefully, easy-to-digest book. You are not alone. Wherever this book is, I am. We are in this together.

What lies within you is the ability to heal yourself, your family and your child. You can do this. Never give up!

IN MEMORY

WITH A HEAVY HEART I dedicate this section of the book to the memory of my mother, Mary Galley. My mom's health took a sharp turn and we lost her in December of 2017, just before Christmas. My mom was one of my greatest allies. She was fierce, brave and the smartest person I have ever known. My mom made sure I went to church and volunteered throughout my life. She and I helped package food and clothing for homeless families every Friday for most of my youth. My mom took me to various protests and we attended the Martin Luther King Day Parade in Denver every year of my childhood that I can remember. She believed in justice, free speech and the God-given right to liberty. She taught me to speak up for the voiceless and to be bold in the face of adversity. She was fearless, and it is an honor to have had her as my mother.

My mom was an exceptional grandmother. She helped me with David's gluten, casein and soy free diet and found ways to make his food taste delicious. She read through mountains of information on autism and spent countless hours helping me piece David's treatment plans together. She was one of my greatest supporters. She was steadfast in her commitment to helping David's health improve and her time, energy and love helped him get to where he is today.

The last few months of her life, my mom was able to spend quality time with Aidan, teaching him our Italian family recipes. She spent hours drawing with Brooks, keeping him company while I attended legislative hearings, Board of Education meetings and working on David's academics. She brought joy to the lives of all my children. She hosted beautiful birthday parties and made sure the holidays were magical for them. She was unwavering in her dedication to my boys and I am forever grateful for her contribution to their lives.

I cannot fully articulate the impact she had on me. I do not have the words to describe what her influence meant to my life other than to say that I am brave because she was brave. I speak up for those who cannot speak for themselves because that is what my mother taught me to do.

In her memory, may we all find our voice; the voice that speaks on behalf of what is just and what is right. In memory of my mom, it is my hope that each person reading this goes out into the world and speaks up for people with autism and those who cannot speak for themselves.

In memory of my mom, may we all persevere against all odds and never give up.

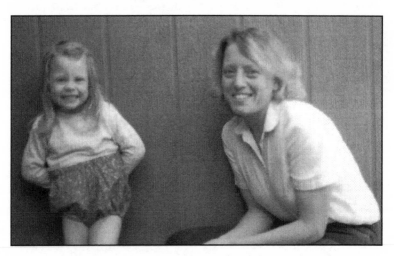

Sarah Carrasco as a young girl with her mother.

NOTES

1. FIRST THINGS FIRST:
TAKE CARE OF YOURSELF

1. Winston S. Churchill, *Never Give In!: The Best of Winston Churchill's Speeches* (New York: Hachette Books, 2004), ii.
2. *Seinfeld*, "The Pitch," Aired September 16, 1992. See: https://www.youtube.com/watch?v=Qw2oM8bTy8M.
3. McCarthy, Jenny. *Louder than Words: A Mother's Journey in Healing Autism*. (New York: Dutton/Penguin, 2008).

2. TAKE THE NEXT FIRST STEP:
GETTING THE DIAGNOSIS OF AUTISM

1. See: http://maryromaniec.com/pdf/danielsstory.pdf.
2. See: http://www.autism.com/pdf/providers/diagnostic_cl _e2.pdf.
3. See: http://www.dramyyasko.com/wp-content/files_flutter /1327512160_9_1_1_8_pdf_02_file.pdf.
4. See: https://www.medmaps.org/.
5. See: https://www.psychiatry.org/File Library/Psychiatrists/ Practice/DSM/APA_DSM-5-Autism-Spectrum-Disorder.pdf.
6. Grandin, Temple. *Thinking in Pictures: And Other Reports from My Life with Autism* (New York: Vintage, 2010), 57, 58, 60.
7. While often attributed to Winston Churchill, the quotation is adapted from an anonymous conversation recorded in an editorial by John Randall Dunn "Binding the Power of Pain," Christian Science Sentinel 45, no. 44 (October 30, 1943).

3. UNDERSTANDING HEALTH INSURANCE AND MEDICAID

1. See: https://www.youtubevNZVV4Ciccg.com/watch? v=.
2. See: https://www.p2pusa.org/p2pusa/SitePages/p2p-support.aspx.
3. See: https://www.medicalhomeportal.org/issue/writing-letters-of-medical-necessity.
4. See: https://www.asha.org/Advocacy/state/States-Specific-Autism-Mandates/.
5. See: https://www.ssa.gov/ssi/text-child-ussi.htm.
6. See: https://secure.ssa.gov/iClaim/dib.
7. See: https://www.familyvoices.org/.
8. See: https://www.icd10codesearch.com.
9. See: http://parenting.blogs.nytimes.com/2012/06/06/be cause-of-katie-children-with-severe-disabilities-can-live-at-home/.
10. See: https://www.medicaid.gov/medicaid/section-1115-de mo/demonstration-and-waiver-list/waivers_faceted.html and http: //medicaidwaiver.org/.
11. See: https://www.ibc-pa.org/.
12. See: http://treatmentplansthatworked.com/.
13. Steven Kosser. *The Issachar Project* (Exton, PA: The Institute for Behavior Change, 2016).
14. See: https://www.thearc.org/what-we-do.
15. See: https://www.thearc.org/find-a-chapter.

4. BIOMEDICAL INTERVENTIONS FOR AUTISM: RECOVERY IS POSSIBLE

1. Jon Pangborn, Ph.D., and Sidney MacDonald Baker, M.D., *Autism: Effective Biomedical Interventions*, vol. 1. (San Diego: Autism Research Institute, 2005).
2. Jon Pangborn, Ph.D., and Sidney MacDonald Baker, M.D., *Autism*.
3. See: https://www.autism.com/index.php/treatment_ratings_ asd.
4. See: https://www.tacanow.org/family-resources/going-gfcfsf -in-10-weeks/.
5. See: https://www.autism.com/ind_atec.
6. See: http://www.klinghardtacademy.com/images/stories/ neurotoxin/NeurotoxinProtocol_Jan06.pdf.

7. See: https://www.recoveringkids.com/getting-started.
8. See: https://biology.uni.edu/sites/default/files/chiroprac tic_education_vs_medical_education.pdf.
9. See: https//www.medmaps.org.
10. Karen DeFelice, *Enzymes for Autism and Other Neurological Conditions*, 3rd ed. (Johnston, IA: ThunderSnow Interactive, 2002).
11. See: http://www.dramyyasko.com/wp-content/files_flutter /1327512160_9_1_1_8_pdf_02_file.pdf.
12. See: http://drsircus.com/autism/magnesium-and-autism/.
13. See: http://www.tacanow.org/family-resources/hbot-for-asd/.
14. See: http://thinkingmomsrevolution.com/wp-content/ uploads/2016/02/TMR-Study-2-Whitepaper-ATEC-Changes- with-the-IonCleanse-by-AMD.pdf.
15. See: https://www.amajordifference.com/?gclid=CMSvxaiu3c8 CFQyIaQodNLoGbw.
16. See: https://www.mammausa.org/.
17. See: http://www.autismone.org/content/dr-john-hicks-med icinal-power-cannabis.
18. See: http://www.oil-testimonials.com/essential-oils/7601/ autism-spectrum-child-chose-his-own-protocol.
19. See: http://www.dnaconnexions.com/.
20. See: http://www.pandasppn.org/SeeingYourFirstChild/.
21. See: http://www.tacanow.org/family-stories/autism-in-past -tense/.
22. Leann Whifften, *A Child's Journey out of Autism: One Family's Story of Living in Hope and Finding a Cure* (Naperville, IL: Source, 2009).
23. See: http://maryromaniec.com/pdf/danielsstory.pdf.
24. See: http://www.tacanow.org/family-resources/more-holi day-survival-tips/.
25. See: http://www.ageofautism.com/2013/07/autism-and-dr- bernie-rimland-harmful-exposures-and-susceptible-children. html.
26. See: http://whale.to/vaccine/synergistic_toxicity_q.html.
27. See: http://healthimpactnews.com/2014/dangerous-doctor -media-vaccine-promoter-has-huge-conflict-of-interest/.
28. See: http://articles.mercola.com/sites/articles/archive/2012 /08/02/merck-flu-vaccine-conflicts.aspx.
29. See: https://vactruth.com/2016/06/25/acetaminophen-and- autism/.

30. See: https://www.youtube.com/watch?v=5F_yj1T8Qu8;
https://www.youtube.com/watch?v=XUORtLSg19E; https://
www.youtube.com/watch?v=nKeOXeGgBY4; and https://
www.youtube.com/ watch?v=8h66beBrEpk.
31. See: http://vaxxedthemovie.com/statement-william-
w-thompson-ph-d-regarding-2004-article-examining-
possibility-relationship-mmr-vaccine-autism/ and https://
sharylattkisson.com/cdc- scientist-we-scheduled-meeting-to-
destroy-vaccine-autism-study-documents/.
32. See: https://sharylattkisson.com/audio-cdc-addresses-all
egations-on-vaccine-autism-link-omission/ and https://
vimeo.com/153178203.
33. See: https://www.cdc.gov/pertussis/downloads/pertusss
urv-report-2014.pdf.
34. See: http://www.abundanthealthlife.com/vaxxed/.
35. See: http://vaxtruth.org/2012/01/aluminum-toxicity-and-a-
primer-on-the-vic/.
36. See: https://www.facebook.com/notes/shawn-siegel/bou
ndaries/903633159664152/.
37. See: https://www.youtube.com/watch?v=buQvtnQ7VXA.
38. See: https://www.youtube.com/watch?v=3wwDPcNdxJQ.
39. See: https://safeminds.org/vaccines-and-autism/correlati on-
between-increases-in-autism-prevalence-and-introduction-of-
new-vaccines/.
40. See: https://www.facebook.com/greenmedinfo/photos/a.17
2939738489.118792.111877548489/10154238595428490
/?type=3.
41. See: https://www.facebook.com/notes/shawn-siegel/a-stroke-
of-the-pen-polio/365804180113722.
42. See: https://www.facebook.com/notes/shawn-siegel/a-stroke-
of-the-pen-polio/365804180113722.
43. See: https://www.facebook.com/notes/shawn-siegel/a-stroke-
of-the-pen-polio/365804180113722.
44. See: https://www.facebook.com/notes/shawn-siegel/a-stroke-
of-the-pen-polio/365804180113722.
45. See: https://www.facebook.com/notes/shawn-siegel/a-stroke-
of-the-pen-polio/365804180113722.
46. See: https://www.facebook.com/notes/shawn-siegel/a-stroke-
of-the-pen-polio/365804180113722.
47. See: http://thinkingmomsrevolution.com/autism-war-fiction-
true-crime/.

48. See: http://thinkingmomsrevolution.com/mrc-5-wi-38-vaccines/.
49. See: http://www.robertfkennedyjr.com/vaccines.html.
50. See: https://www.washingtonpost.com/news/storyline/wp/2015/01/30/mississippi-yes-mississippi-has-the-nations-best-child-vaccination-rate-heres-why.
51. See: http://www.ageofautism.com/2014/09/mercury-sim psonwood-2000-and-an-elementary-cover-up.html.
52. See: http://sharylattkisson.com/fact-check-false-reports-c laiming-calif-measles-outbreak-killed-children/.
53. See: http://naturalsociety.com/mit-scientist-glyphosate-to -cause-autism-in-50-of-children-by-2025/.
54. See: http://naturalsociety.com/mit-scientist-glyphosate-to -cause-autism-in-50-of-children-by-2025/.

5. AUTISM-RELATED THERAPIES AND INTERVENTIONS

1. Andre Masse, CSE, "Beatitudes for Friends of Disabled Children," *NAMR Quarterly*, 1968. See: https://www.autismspeaks.org/sites/default/files/docs/the_beatitudes_of_the_exceptional_child.pdf.
2. See: http://www.sensoryprocessingdisorderparentsupport.com/ wilbarger-brushing-compressions.php.
3. See: https://www.facebook.com/sarah.carrasco.56/videos/vb.1300900337/10209566291016386/?type=2&theater.
4. See: http://www.ageofautism.com/2014/08/journal-exercise-47-autobiographical-incident-7-11-14.html.
5. See: http://www.ageofautism.com/2014/08/journal-exercise-47-autobiographical-incident-7-11-14.html.
6. See: http://www.ageofautism.com/2014/08/journal-exercise-47-autobiographical-incident-7-11-14.html.
7. See: http://www.ageofautism.com/2014/08/journal-exercise-47-autobiographical-incident-7-11-14.html.
8. See: http://www.tacanow.org/family-resources/helping-nonverbal-kids-to-communicate/.
9. See: http://www.autismtreatmentcenter.org/contents/prog rams_and_services/startup_qanda.php.
10. See: http://www.users.qwest.net/~tbharris/prt.htm.
11. See: https://www.socialthinking.com/LandingPages/Mission.
12. See: http://www.musictherapy.org/assets/1/7/MT_Autism _2012.pdf.

13. See: http://www.musictherapy.org/assets/1/7/MT_
Autism_2012.pdf.
14. See: http://www.halo-soma.org/learning_methodology.php.
15. See: http://www.halo-soma.org/learning_methodology.ph
p?sess_id=561a4ec61f90eaa5f51d7634baf3cd72.
16. See: http://www.thetappingsolution.com/what-is-eft-
tapping/.
17. See: http://www.annemevans.com/.

6. EDUCATION

1. See: http://www.masters-education.com/masters-in-special
-education/.
2. See: https://disabilitylawco.org/news/third-edition-every
day-guide-special-education-law/01-31-2015
3. See: http://www.wrightslaw.com/.
4. Lisa Ackerman, *Autism Journey Guide: A Starting Point for
Parents Facing Autism* (Costa Mesa, CA: TACA (Talk about
Curing Autism), 2008).
5. See: https://www.facebook.com/sarah.carrasco.56/
videos/vb.1300900337/10209566291016386/?ty
pe=2&theater and http://www.wildwoodonline.org/
uploads/2/5/9/4/25947660/understanding_autism.pdf.
6. See: http://www.touchmath.com/.
7. See: http://www.starfall.com/.
8. See: https://www.mwl-law.com/wp-content/uploads/2013
/03/LAWS-ON-RECORDING-CONVERSATIONS-CHART.pdf.
9. Dale Carnegie, *How to Win Friends & Influence People*
(Sydney: HarperCollins Australia, 2017).
10. See: http://www2.ed.gov/about/offices/list/ocr/docs/how
to.html.

7. PREPARING YOUR CHILD FOR ADOLESCENCE AND ADULTHOOD

1. See: www.thereasonijump.com
2. See: http://www.pecsusa.com/pecs.php.
3. See: http://www.tacanow.org/?s=communication.
4. See: http://www.tacanow.org/family-resources/teens-with-
asd-life-skills/.
5. See: http://marquettestrengthsindex.com/wp/.

6. See: https://www.docguide.com/puzzling-seizures-could-be-related-autoimmune-condition.
7. See: http://www.tacanow.org/family-resources/teens-with-asd-puberty/.
8. See: http://www.epilepsy.com/learn/triggers-seizures/nutri tional-deficiencies.
9. See: http://www.tacanow.org/family-resources/teens-with -asd-puberty/.
10. See: https://www.tacanow.org/family-resources/teens-with -asd-puberty/.

8. YOUR NEW LIFE

1. See: http://www.tacanow.org/family-resources/divorce-advice-for-special-needs-families/.
2. See: https://www.huffingtonpost.com/m-lin/special-needs -parents_b_1338169.html.
3. See: https://www.ada.gov/t3hilght.htm.
4. See: http://www.kellybroganmd.com.
5. See: http://www.safewise.com/blog/10-wearable-safety-gps-devices-kids/.
6. See: http://nationalautismassociation.org/big-red-safety-box/naas-big-red-safety-teacher-toolkit-now-available/.

9. LEGAL CONSIDERATIONS

1. See: http://www.mangusfinance.com.
2. See: http://www.ablenrc.org/about/what-are-able-accounts.
3. See: http://www.ca-specialneedstrusts.com/conservatorship. htm.
4. See: https://www.ada.gov/qandaeng.htm.
5. See: https://www.ada.gov/qandaeng.htm.
6. See: https://www.ada.gov/qandaeng.htm.
7. See: https://www.nij.gov/topics/victims-victimization/ Documents/violent-victimization-twg-2015-browne-demyan-agha.pdf.
8. See: https://www.nij.gov/topics/victims-victimization/ Documents/violent-victimization-twg-2015-browne-demyan-agha.pdf.
9. See: http://www.thearc.org/document.doc?id=3664.
10. See: http://www.thearc.org/document.doc?id=3664.

11. See: http://www.thearc.org/document.doc?id=3664.
12. See: https://www.thearc.org/document.doc?id=3669.
13. See: https://www.thearc.org/document.doc?id=3669.
14. See: https://www.thearc.org/document.doc?id=3669.

10. LIFE WITH AUTISM

1. See: http://www.ageofautism.com/2014/08/journal-exercise-47-autobiographical-incident-7-11-14.html.
2. See: https://www.autism.com/advocacy_grandin.
3. See: https://www.autism.com/advocacy_grandin.
4. See: https://www.youtubevNZVV4Ciccg.com/watch?v= and https://www.youtube.com/watch?v=KmDGvquzn2k.
5. Jenny McCarthy, *Louder Than Words*.
6. Naoki Higashida, *The Reason I Jump: The Inner Voice of a Thirteen-Year-Old Boy with Autism*, trans. K. A. Yoshida and David Mitchell (New York: Random House, 2016). See: http://thereasonijump.com/.
7. Tyler McNamer, *Population One: Autism, Adversity, and the Will to Succeed* (Lake Placid, NY: Aviva Publishing, 2013). See: https://www.kickstarter.com/projects/tylermcnamer/population-one-autism-adversity-and-the-will-to-su-0.
8. Arthur Fleischmann with Carly Fleischmann, *Carly's Voice: Breaking through Autism* (New York: Simon & Schuster, 2012). See: https://www.youtube.com/watch?v=xMBzJleeOno.
9. Arthur Fleishmann, *Carly's Voice*. See: https://www.youtube.com/watch?v=xMBzJleeOno.
10. Naoki Higashida, *The Reason I Jump*, xv, emphasis in original.

ACKNOWLEDGMENTS

I ALWAYS THANK GOD FIRST. It is from Him all blessings flow. In the darkest days, it was my faith that kept the light inside me burning; although dim at times, the light and love of God has been my source of comfort through the worst of times. I am thankful to God for all things; currently, I make just enough money to pay our bills and buy food. There is no extra money. Somehow, we always have enough to eat, clothes, the kids have (arguably too many) toys, a roof over our heads, and when I need money for David, things always fall into place and I find a way to cover the expenses.

I believe that God has called me to serve people with autism; to protect, honor, and advocate for his most precious children. It is an honor to be called for this purpose; the trials and tribulations I have experienced along the way have made me sharper, stronger, and fiercer than I ever thought I could be. It was through these difficult experiences that I gained the skills and knowledge necessary to advocate for people with autism. For this, I am truly grateful.

I would like to thank my publisher, Dr. Andy McCabe of City Bear Press. I knew you were the right fit when you told me you had written a book titled *How Women Will Change the World.* I started writing this book several years ago and submitted hundreds of requests to agents and small publishing houses to no avail. Despite the disappointment, inherently I knew that the right publisher would have to be someone who valued and believed in the power of women.

Your book highlights the most valuable lessons women can learn. Although *How Women Will Change the World* is fiction, the lessons learned from the stories are absolute truths. Women can be hypercritical of themselves, and it can stifle their path to enlightenment. It is when women believe in ourselves that we harness the God-given power of intuition. It is with this divine power that we will change the world. Your book asserts that the time has come for the divine feminine awakening, that the time of men ruling the world and creating perpetual war needs to be balanced out by the peace only women can bring to the earth. You are correct in your assertion; what the world needs to heal is the divine feminine awakening. Good men see the value in women. Thank you for being such a good man.

The time I have spent on the phone with you, talking about the book and the state of the world has been incredibly healing and encouraging for me. I consider you one of my dearest friends. Thank you for believing in me.

I want to thank my dear friend Phil Silberman who helped me edit this book (before it went to the editor). While I am a good writer, your edits make my words shine. Your input has been valuable in ways I can never fully articulate. More than anything, your willingness to help me, knowing I could not pay you, means the world to me; your kindness has helped restore my faith in people. Your words of praise and you believing in me helped me to heal from old wounds. Sometimes a kind word can go a long way. Thank you for your time, advice, and kind words.

I want to give a special thank you to Mary Romaniec. You basically saved our lives so...thank you. I can't bring myself to think about where David would be if it were not for your article. You helped save his life, and that is a debt I can never repay. Thank you for being you. Your concern for the world around you has inspired me to tell my story and speak my truth; you taught me that my story can help heal others who are in a similar circumstance. Your courage has given me courage. Thank you for being a good friend and such a wonderful advocate for our kids. You are forever a part of our story.

I would be remiss to not thank my family. Mom and Dad, neither one of you has had it particularly easy and yet you maintain a sense of optimism and hope that is admirable. You live as Christians should live. You are some of the only people I know who will take in those who are struggling and give them shelter. The last few years have been tough for me, and I appreciate you being there when I need you. You are two of the smartest, toughest, and most resilient people I know. It is an honor to be your daughter. I love you both very much.

To my sister, Chris, thank you for your help along the way. You see our struggles and do your best to relieve them. Your help with the kids' school clothes, shoes, boots, coats, and giving them money for Target is much appreciated. When I needed a new dishwasher, and lost all my keys, you helped me when I needed you most. These past few years have been difficult in a way I can't explain. Thank you for relieving me of burdens I could not have borne alone.

To my sister, Liz, and my brother-in-law, Jerry, thank you for always buying the kids such nice Christmas and birthday presents. I cannot always afford to buy them the things they want, and I appreciate you giving them the things I can't always give them. Thank you for making them feel special.

One of the people who helped us the most was David's Certified Occupational Therapy Assistant (COTA), Cindy. Out of desperation, I prayed/cried/begged God for mercy when things were at their worst; God answered my prayers by sending Cindy to us. Thank you, Cindy. If not for your dedication and perseverance, David would not be where he is today. It took years to get him to hold a pencil and write his name, yet you stuck by him. He hit, kicked, bit, and scratched you, and you refused to give up on him. His fine and gross motor skills would not be where they are today if not for you. You have given me articles and resources that changed the course of our lives. You stayed when most people left. Thank you for staying.

My friends have been my saving grace through all of this. I am fortunate enough to have had many of the same friends for over twenty years. Some of them visited me when I could not leave the house with David. They came to me on my birthdays knowing I couldn't leave the house. They were my life raft when I felt like I was drowning. Thank you, guys, for saving me, even when you didn't realize you were.

My Facebook friends have changed the trajectory of my life. I am thankful for each of my fearless, outspoken, brilliant and unabashedly honest warrior friends. You have helped me heal David when no expert could. You have guided, mentored, encouraged and inspired me. It is an honor you call you my friends. You are the change the world so desperately needs.

My Grandma Olga was my very best friend. I love her as much today as I did when she passed twenty years ago. My Grandma was brave, tough, kind, and fiercely protective of her family. She loved me unconditionally and taught me to love and respect God. When I start to feel overwhelmed or afraid, I ask myself, "What would Grandma do?" And the answer is always the same; she would be brave, unafraid, and she would defend her children with the will of an army. Thank you, Grandma Olga; the best parts of me came from you. Until we meet again....

Lastly, I want to give thanks to my children. David, you have fundamentally changed me for the better. It is out of my love for you and my God-given duty to protect you that I have become the person I am today. Thank you for being such a good example for the rest of us. Your kind heart, gentle spirit, and forgiving nature are an inspiration. I am continuously in awe of you. Thank you for giving my life meaning. Aidan, you are the best brother a kid could ask for. You are always there to support David and, according to him, you are "the best brother and friend." Before you were born, I prayed for someone to come into my life who was positive, kind, and who would love me unconditionally. God sent me you. Thank you for being a rock in our family. You have endured the hardships in our life with grace and dignity. You have been a source of comfort to me and the voice of reason when I needed it most. You are an activist in your own right; justice has always been paramount in your thinking, and I am immensely proud of you for it. You are wise beyond your years. Thank you for everything you do for David and our family. And finally, my little Brooks. You are still too young to realize the complexities of what life has been for us, and for that I am thankful. Your strong will combined with a kind heart will serve the world well. At four years old, you have the tenacity of a hundred men; I know you will use it for good. You are already protective of David and your family; the love of family can drive social change. Your strong will can change the world. I love you very much, son. God bless you, my angels. Thank you for giving my life purpose and meaning.

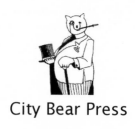

City Bear Press

Publishing Books that Will Change the World

Our mission is to publish books that will have the potential to make a real difference in our world. We are a publishing house without walls which allows us to pay our authors far more than conventional brick and mortar companies.

We publish a limited number of books each year. If you have a manuscript that you think meets our criteria, contact us through our website: www.citybearpress.com and forward your book title and contact information.

Books by City Bear Press

How Women Will Change the World
by Dr. Andy McCabe

The Autism Help Book
by Sarah Carrasco

Made in the USA
San Bernardino, CA
02 August 2018